SCAM

SO-CALLED ALTERNATIVE MEDICINE

Edzard Ernst

SOCIETAS
essays in political
& cultural criticism

imprint-academic.com

Published in the UK by
Imprint Academic Ltd., PO Box 200, Exeter EX5 5YX, UK

Distributed in the USA by
Ingram Book Company,
One Ingram Blvd., La Vergne, TN 37086, USA

ISBN 9781845409708 paperback

A CIP catalogue record for this book is available from the
British Library and US Library of Congress

To Danielle

Contents

Preface

I should perhaps start with a warning: this book might unsettle you. If you are a true believer in so-called alternative medicine (SCAM), you may find the things I am about to tell you disturbing. My book was not written for true believers. In my experience, they often are emotionally or intellectually unable to rationalise and to change their minds. Any attempt at opening their eyes and making them think critically might therefore be a waste of time.

This book was written for everyone who has an interest in SCAM and is open to considering the evidence. Yet it is not a guidebook that tells you which SCAM can be employed for what condition. It is a compilation of 50 essays about SCAM in more general terms. I ordered them loosely under seven headings and have tried to write them in such a way that they can be read independently. This necessitated a certain amount of repetition of crucial themes which, I hope, is forgivable. My main aim in publishing this book is to stimulate your ability to think critically about healthcare in general and, of course, about SCAM in particular.

The book is based on my 25 years of research in SCAM. It quotes numerous investigations by my team and by other researchers. It also discusses many recently published examples of pseudo-science, misleading information and unethical SCAM-promotion. The text avoids technical language and should be easily understood by anyone. The 'glossary' at the end of the book provides additional explanations of more complex issues and terminology. Throughout the book, I use hints of irony, touches of satire, and sometimes even a degree of exaggeration. This makes certain points clearer and might even make you smile from time to time.

Working on this book was great fun, and I sincerely hope you find the result both informative and entertaining.

Chapter 1

Introduction

> *Usually and fitly, the presence of an introduction is held to imply that there is something of consequence and importance to be introduced.* – Arthur Machen

Why do I call it SCAM? Why not just 'alternative medicine' or one of the many other possible names for it? [BOX 1] Mainly because, whatever it is, it is it is <u>not</u> an alternative:

- if a therapy does not work, it cannot be an alternative to medicine;
- if a therapy does work, it does not belong to alternative medicine but to medicine.

Therefore, I think that so-called alternative medicine or SCAM is not a bad term to use.

My years in SCAM research can be divided into three periods. The first was characterised by defining the aims of my research, assembling a team, getting the infrastructure sorted and starting a research programme. From the very beginning, I had made it clear that I needed to be sceptical and was determined not to promote SCAM but to critically evaluate it and produce good science on the way. In my memoir,[1] I describe the moment when I expressed this publicly for the very first time:

---

[1] http://books.imprint.co.uk/book/?gcoi=71157100246620, also available at https://www.amazon.co.uk/Scientist-Wonderland-Searching-Finding-Trouble/dp/1845407776.

As my new position was the first chair of its kind, the university administrators had decided to organise a press conference... In this particular instance, not only I, but also Sir Maurice Laing (who had endowed the chair), and finally, the Vice Chancellor of the university were to make brief statements, after which the journalists would have an opportunity to quiz us. As alternative medicine was a controversial topic, we tried to play it safe: the Vice Chancellor praised the generosity of Sir Maurice and spoke of the unique opportunity his endowment would offer for both the university and the field of complementary medicine, as well as of the University's good fortune in finding an experienced professor to tackle this difficult but important task. For his part, Sir Maurice told the audience of his deep conviction that rigorous research was the best way to reveal the true value of the treatments that he and his wife had repeatedly found helpful. Then it was my turn. I outlined my professional background, explained what rigorous research in alternative medicine would entail and where it might take us. When I had finished, one journalist in the front row raised his hand: 'What will you do, Prof Ernst, when your medical colleagues turn out to be sceptical about alternative medicine?' Shooting from the hip, I answered: 'I am not too worried about that, because I intend to be more sceptical than they are.'

Realising how controversial some of our research might become, I made a conscious effort during this first period to keep clear of disputes and to avoid the limelight. I wanted to first do my 'homework', analyse the evidence, produce own results and be quite sure of my own position before engaging in any public debates. During this time, my team and I published almost exclusively in medical journals, lectured to medical audiences and generally kept a low a public profile. [BOX 2]

The second period of my involvement in SCAM was characterised by yet more research and the realisation that, occasionally, it would be necessary to 'stick my head out' and stand up publicly for our findings. The evidence generated not just by our own research but by scientists across the planet more and more clearly showed that:

- few forms of SCAM seemed to work,
- many seemed not to do more good than harm,
- and most SCAMs were so under-researched that it was impossible to tell.

In our 'Desktop Guide to Complementary and Alternative Medicine'[2] we evaluated around 700 treatment/condition pairs and determined the percentage that was supported by sound evidence. The resulting figure was 7.4%.[3] Put simply, only about 7 of 100 SCAMs seemed to be based on good evidence and could be recommended for routine use. Analysing the findings of another book, *Natural Standard*,[4] in a similar fashion produced comparable results. The authors of this volume had graded 507 therapy/condition pairs. Of these, 49 were supported by 'strong scientific evidence'. The percentage of evidence-based SCAMs thus amounted to 9.7%. The two figures (7.4 and 9.7%) are strikingly similar, yet I fear that both were gross over-estimates. They were derived from books which focused on SCAMs for which there was at least some evidence. Had all SCAMs been included indiscriminately, the resulting percentages would certainly have been much smaller.

Surely this type of information was important for consumers, I felt. In the realm of SCAM, the public often make decisions without consulting even a single healthcare professional. Therefore, they need accurate and reliable information regardless of whether the evidence was positive or negative. Realising this, I began publishing in the daily papers,

---

[2] https://www.amazon.co.uk/d/cka/Desktop-Guide-Complementary-Alternative-Medicine-Evidence-Based-Approach/0723432074/ref=sr_1_4?s=books&ie=UTF8&qid=1499948538&sr=1-4&keywords=ernst+edzard.

[3] https://www.ncbi.nlm.nih.gov/pubmed/?term=Ernst+E.+How+much+of+CAM+is+based+on+research+evidence%3F+eCAM+2009%3B+doi%3A10.1093%2Fecam%2Fnep044.

[4] https://www.amazon.co.uk/Natural-Standard-Herb-Supplement-Guide/dp/032307295X/ref=sr_1_1?s=books&ie=UTF8&qid=1499948788&sr=1-1&keywords=Natural+Standard.

lecturing regularly to lay audiences, and addressing the public in any way that seemed appropriate.

By the late 1990s, several independent analyses had shown that my team had become the most productive research unit in SCAM worldwide,[5] and we started receiving requests from scientists across the globe to join us. Many of those individuals later went back to their home countries to occupy key positions in research. Our concept of critical evaluation thus spread around the world. Amongst the ~90 staff who have worked for me during the last 25 years, we had many enthusiastic and gifted scientists. I owe thanks to all of them.

The third phase of my involvement in SCAM is still ongoing; it started after I retired from my Exeter post in 2012/ 2013 (I officially retired in 2012 but was subsequently re-employed by my university for half a year). Now I had more time and freedom for reflection, and consequently my attitude towards SCAM became more sceptical. I started writing a regular blog (where many of the ideas for this book were first generated), published several books,[6, 7, 8] and no longer had to fear getting reprimanded by my peers for not always adhering to the rules of political correctness. In 2015, I was awarded the John Maddox Prize for standing up for science,[9] and in 2017 I received the Ockham Award[10] for the work on my blog (http://edzardernst.com/).

Some of my critics like to claim that I never did anything but debunk SCAM. This is certainly not true. In 2008, I even published a summary of all the SCAMs that, according to our analyses, were based on sound evidence.[11] What is true,

5   https://www.ncbi.nlm.nih.gov/pubmed/12442823.
6   https://www.amazon.co.uk/Scientist-Wonderland-Searching-Finding-Trouble/dp/1845407776.
7   http://www.hive.co.uk/Product/Professor-Edzard-Ernst/Homeopathy---The-Undiluted-Facts--Including-a-Comprehensive-A-Z-Lexicon/19719982.
8   Ernst E., Smith K., *More Harm Than Good? The moral maze of complementary and alternative medicine*, Springer, Heidelberg (in press).
9   http://senseaboutscience.org/activities/2015-john-maddox-prize/.
10   https://www.skeptic.org.uk/published/the-ockham-awards/.
11   https://www.ncbi.nlm.nih.gov/pubmed/18318982.

however, is that I prefer rigorous science to wishful thinking, a stance that many SCAM proponents find hard to accept. The disappointment of SCAM enthusiasts had been palpable virtually from the start. In my memoir,[12] I describe the moment when I first realised this:

> ...I had accepted an invitation to address this meeting packed with about 100 proponents of alternative medicine. I felt that their enthusiasm and passion were charming but, no matter whom I talked to, there seemed to be little or no understanding of the role of science in all this. A child-like naïvety pervaded this audience: alternative practitioners and their supporters seemed a bit like children playing 'doctor and patient'. The language, the rituals and the façade were all more or less in place, but somehow they seemed strangely detached from reality. They passionately wanted to promote alternative medicine, while I, with equal passion, wanted to conduct good science. The two aims were profoundly different, but I nevertheless managed to convince myself that they were not irreconcilable, and that we would manage to combine our passions and create something worthwhile, perhaps even ground-breaking... Science, I pointed out, generates progress through asking critical questions and through testing hypotheses. Alternative medicine would either be shown by good science to be of value, or it would turn out to be little more than a passing fad. The endowment of the Laing chair represented an important milestone on the way towards the impartial evaluation of alternative medicine, and surely this would be in the best interest of all parties concerned... My audience, however, was not impressed. When I had finished, there was a stunned silence. Finally someone shouted angrily from the back row: 'How did they dare to appoint a doctor to this chair?' I was blindsided by this and did not quite

---

[12] https://www.amazon.co.uk/Scientist-Wonderland-Searching-Finding-Trouble/dp/1845407776.

understand. What had prompted this reaction? What did these people expect? Did they think my qualifications were not good enough? Why were they upset by the appointment of a doctor? Who else, in their view, might be better equipped to conduct medical research?

Their hope of me becoming an uncritical promotor of SCAM has been frustrated ever since. This book, I am afraid, will be yet another disappointment to them.

BOX 1
Common names for SCAM

- ALTERNATIVE MEDICINE is an umbrella term for therapeutic and diagnostic modalities employed as a replacement of conventional modalities.
- COMPLEMENTATY MEDICINE is an umbrella term for modalities usually employed as an adjunct to conventional healthcare.
- COMPLEMENTARY AND ALTERNATIVE MEDICINE (CAM) combines both expressions because the same SCAM modality can often be employed either as a replacement of or an add-on to conventional medicine.
- DISPROVEN MEDICINE is an umbrella term for treatments that have been shown not to work.
- FRINGE MEDICINE is the term formerly used for alternative medicine.
- HOLISTIC MEDICINE is healthcare that emphasises whole patient care.
- INTEGRATED MEDICINE describes the use of treatments that allegedly incorporate 'the best of both worlds', i.e. the best of SCAM and conventional healthcare.
- INTEGRATIVE MEDICINE is the same as above but more common in the UK.
- NATURAL MEDICINE is healthcare exclusively employing the means provided by nature for treating disease.
- QUACKERY is the deliberate misinterpretation of the ability of a treatment or diagnostic technique to treat or diagnose disease.
- TRADITIONAL MEDICINE is healthcare that has been in use before the scientific era (the assumption often is that such treatments have stood the test of time).
- UNCONVENTIONAL MEDICINE is healthcare not normally used in conventional medicine (this would include off-label use of drugs, for instance, and therefore is not a good term for SCAM).
- UNORTHODOX MEDICINE is a term for healthcare that is not normally used in orthodox medicine.
- UNPROVEN MEDICINE is healthcare that lacks scientific proof (many conventional therapies fall in this category too).

BOX 2
Essential facts about SCAM

- SCAM includes a diverse array of therapeutic, preventative and diagnostic modalities. Some of the most popular are acupuncture, aromatherapy, applied kinesiology, chiropractic, energy healing, herbal medicine, homeopathy, iridology, massage therapy, reflexology.
- SCAM is currently popular; 30–70% of the general population have used at least one type of SCAM during the preceding year; for patient populations, there figures usually are considerably higher.
- The basic assumptions of many forms of SCAM are not plausible, i.e. they contradict the laws of nature as we understand them today.
- The effectiveness of most forms of SCAM is unproven, in some cases even disproven.
- Contrary to many claims by SCAM providers, most forms of SCAM are not free of risks.
- Regardless of these concerns, SCAM is currently becoming widely accepted by the medical profession and by health politicians.
- Powerful lobby-groups promote SCAM and advocate its further integration into conventional healthcare.

Chapter 2

The Basics

Better to light a candle than curse the darkness. — *Chinese Proverb*

2.1. Evidence and Experience

Many people strongly believe in SCAM. Others are just as reverently opposed to it. The two camps tend to engage in endless discussions about who is right and who is wrong. Who is telling the truth and who is promoting falsehoods? The only way to find out is to critically assess the evidence.

Clinicians and their patients often feel that their daily experience holds valuable information about the efficacy or effectiveness of the therapy they administer or receive (efficacy means a therapy works under ideal conditions; effectiveness means it works under everyday conditions). If a patient gets better, they assume this to be the result of the treatment, especially if the experience is repeated. For many clinicians, experience is more meaningful than evidence. While I do sympathise with this notion (I have been a clinician for many years), I nevertheless doubt that they are correct.

Two events — the treatment administered by the clinician and the improvement experienced by the patient — that follow each other in time are not necessarily causally related. Correlation is not the same as causation! The crowing of the cock is not the cause of the sun rising in the morning. In other words, we ought to consider other possible explanations for a patient's improvement after receiving a therapy.

Even the most superficial glance at the possibilities discloses several options.

- The natural history of the condition: most conditions get better, even if they are not treated at all.
- The regression towards the mean: over time, outliers tend to return to the middle.
- The placebo effect: expectation and conditioning affects how we feel.
- Concomitant treatments: patients often take more than one treatment, and it can be impossible to say which worked and which did not.
- Social desirability: patients tend to claim they feel better simply to please their therapist.

These are just some of the most obvious factors that can determine the clinical outcome in such a way that even ineffective treatments can appear to be effective. What follows is undeniable and plausible to scientists, yet intensely counter-intuitive to clinicians who are convinced of the value of their interventions: the prescribed treatment is only one of many factors that affect the clinical outcome.

Clinicians frequently disagree with this line of thinking and produce several counter-arguments:

1) My patient's improvement was so prompt that it must have been caused by my treatment (this notion is not convincing because placebo effects can be just as prompt and direct).

2) I have seen this so many times that it cannot be a coincidence (some clinicians are very caring, charismatic and empathetic; they will thus regularly generate powerful placebo responses).

3) A study with several thousand patients has shown that 70% of them improved after receiving that treatment (such high response rates are typical, even for ineffective treatments, if patient expectation was high).

4) Surely chronic conditions don't suddenly get better; my treatment therefore cannot be a placebo (this is incorrect, most chronic conditions eventually improve, if only temporarily).

5) I had a patient with cancer who received this treatment and was cured (perhaps the patient also received conventional treatments; and, in rare instances, even cancer patients show spontaneous remissions).

6) I have tried the treatment myself and had a positive outcome (clinicians are not immune to the multifactorial nature of the perceived clinical response).

7) Even children and animals respond very well to my treatment; surely, they are not prone to placebo effects (animals can be conditioned to respond; then there is, of course, the natural history of the disease, as mentioned above; and finally, we know about the 'placebo effect by proxy' where the pet owner or parent (rather than the patient) respond to the placebo).

Does that mean that clinical experience is useless? Certainly not, but when it comes to therapeutic effectiveness, clinical experience can be no replacement for evidence. Experience is invaluable for a lot of other things, but, at best, it provides us with a hint and never a proof of effectiveness. Over-reliance on experience can easily generate misleading impressions and bogus claims. [BOX 3]

What, then, is reliable evidence? Essentially, we need to know what would have happened, if our patients had not received the treatment in question. We need to create a situation where we can account for all the factors that might determine the outcome other than the treatment *per se*. Ideally, we would need an experiment where two groups of patients are exposed to the full range of factors, while the only difference is that one group does receive the treatment, while the other one does not. And this is precisely the model of a controlled clinical trial.

Controlled clinical trials are designed to minimise all possible sources of uncertainty about what might have been the cause of the observed effect. As the name indicates, they have a control group which means that, at the end of the treatment period, we can compare the effects of the treatment in question with those of another intervention, a placebo or no treatment at all.

Many different variations of the controlled trial exist so that the exact design can be adapted to the requirements of the treatment under scrutiny and to the specific research question at hand. The overriding principle is, however, always the same: we want to make sure that we can reliably determine whether it was truly the treatment that caused the clinical outcome.

Causality is the key in all of this; and here lies the crucial difference between clinical experience and a clinical trial. What clinicians witness in their daily practice can have myriad causes; what scientists observe in a well-designed study is most likely caused by the treatment *per se*. The latter is evidence, while the former is not.

Yet nobody would claim that clinical trials are perfect. They can have many flaws and have rightly been criticised for a plethora of inherent limitations. Despite all their shortcomings, they are far superior to any other method for determining the efficacy of medical interventions; they represent, so to speak, the worst kind of evidence, except for all other options.

There are many reasons why a clinical trial might generate an incorrect result. We therefore should, whenever possible, avoid relying on the findings of one single study. Independent replications are usually required before we can be sure. Unfortunately, the findings of these replications do not always confirm the results of the previous study. Whenever we are faced with conflicting results, it is tempting to cherry-pick those studies which seem to confirm our prior belief—tempting but very wrong. To arrive at the most reliable conclusion about the effectiveness of any treatment, we need to consider the totality of the reliable evidence. This goal is best achieved by conducting what experts call a 'systematic review'.

In a systematic review, we assess the quality and quantity of the available evidence, synthesise the findings and arrive at an overall verdict about the effectiveness of the treatment in question. Systematic reviews constitute, according to a broad consensus of experts, the best available evidence for or against the effectiveness of any treatment.

Why is evidence important? In a way, this question has already been answered: only with reliable evidence can we tell with any degree of certainty that it was the treatment *per se* — and not any of the other factors mentioned above — that caused the clinical outcome after a treatment. Only if we have such evidence can we be sure about cause and effect. And only then can we make sure that patients receive the best possible treatments currently available.

But, in the realm of SCAM, there are many who say that causality does not matter all that much. What is important, they claim, is to help the patient. And if it was a placebo effect that did the trick, who cares? There are many reasons why this assumption is wrong. To mention just one: it would be a fallacy to assume that we need a placebo treatment to generate a placebo response. If a clinician administers an efficacious therapy (one that generates benefit beyond placebo) with compassion, time, empathy and understanding, she will generate a placebo response **plus** a response to the therapy administered. It follows that merely administering a placebo is less than optimal; in fact, it usually means cheating the patient of the effect of an efficacious therapy.

BOX 3
Examples of bogus claims in SCAM

- Homeopaths claim to be able to treat any condition with their 'high potency remedies'.
- Chiropractors insist that spinal manipulation improves health and well-being.
- Energy healers state that their 'vital energy' improves symptoms.
- SCAM practitioners claim that they treat the root cause of diseases.
- Acupuncturists say that rebalancing yin and yang affects health.
- Naturopaths claim they can detox our bodies.
- Entrepreneurs promote their unproven products as cures for diabetes, cancer, etc.
- Academics teach the benefits of homeopathy to students.
- Homeopaths claim that their remedies are effective alternatives to vaccinations.

2.2. More Good than Harm?

The value of any therapy is not determined by its benefits alone, but by the balance between its risks and benefits. Some treatments, for instance, are very risky (e.g. chemotherapy), yet they can still be enormously valuable when they save lives. Many SCAM proponents stress the dangers of conventional treatments, while claiming that SCAMs are more or less risk-free. This notion, however, is sadly not true.

When discussing the risks of SCAM, I find it usually helpful to divide them into two broad categories:

1. direct risks of the intervention itself,

2. indirect risks usually due to the advice given by SCAM practitioners.

Indirect risks

The indirect risks are often neglected but they are, in fact, often more important than the direct risks. They include forfeiting or delaying effective treatments due to following advice from SCAM providers. Several investigations have recently highlighted this important problem.

A study[1] from Singapore, for example, investigated the impact of SCAM-use on the initiation of disease-modifying anti-rheumatic drugs (DMARD). Data were collected prospectively from 180 patients with arthritis. The results showed that SCAM-users initiated DMARD almost half a year later than non-users. These findings are akin to the results of a recent study with 340 Malaysian cancer patients where SCAM-use was associated with delays in presentation, diagnosis and treatment of breast cancer.[2]

Delaying effective treatments is bad enough, but forfeiting potentially life-saving therapies is clearly worse. An investigation of 281 patients with various types of cancers who chose SCAM as a sole treatment showed that SCAM-use was associated with substantially greater risk of early death compared with conventional cancer treatments. The authors

---

[1]   https://www.ncbi.nlm.nih.gov/pubmed/28524619.
[2]   https://www.ncbi.nlm.nih.gov/pubmed/28448541.

concluded that *SCAM utilization for curable cancer… is associated with greater risk of death.*[3]

But perhaps actual case histories are more convincing than statistics. Turkish surgeons, for instance, reported two cases of middle-aged women suffering from malignant breast masses.[4] The patients experienced serious complications in response to self-prescribed use of SCAMs to treat their condition in lieu of evidence-based medical treatments. In both cases, the use and/or inappropriate application of SCAMs promoted the progression of malignant fungating lesions in the breast. The first patient sought medical assistance upon development of an open lesion, 7–8 cm in diameter and involving 1/3 of the breast, with a palpable mass of 5×6 cm immediately beneath the wound. The second patient sought medical assistance after developing a wide, bleeding, ulcerous area with patchy necrotic tissue that comprised 2/3 of the breast and had a 10×6 cm palpable mass under the affected area. The surgeons concluded that *it is critical that the public is informed about the potential problems of self-treating wounds such as breast ulcers and masses. Additionally, campaigns are needed to increase awareness of the risks and life-threatening potential of using non-evidence-based medical therapies exclusively.*

The factors contributing to such indirect risks of SCAM include:

- Most SCAM practitioners are not trained to responsibly advise patients with serious conditions.
- They often overestimate what their therapy can achieve.
- The patients of SCAM practitioners are frequently desperate and ready to believe even the tallest tales.
- SCAM practitioners often have an important conflict of interest—to make a living, they want to treat as

---

[3]   https://academic.oup.com/jnci/article-abstract/110/1/djx145/4064136/
       Use-of-Alternative-Medicine-for-Cancer-and-Its?redirectedFrom=fulltext.
[4]   https://www.ncbi.nlm.nih.gov/pubmed/25050141.

many patients as possible and are therefore not motivated to refer them to more suitable care.

- They tend to be in denial about the risks of their treatments.
- They are not educated to understand the full complexities of life-threatening diseases.
- As a result, they frequently misguide their patients to make tragically wrong choices.
- In most countries, the regulators turn a blind eye to such problems.

Direct risks

The direct risks of SCAM obviously depend on the specific therapy under investigation. Examples include:

- Stroke after chiropractic or osteopathic spinal manipulations;
- Pneumothorax after acupuncture;
- Liver damage due to herbal medicine.

As there is no monitoring system of adverse effects of SCAM equivalent to those that are mandatory in conventional healthcare, nobody knows for sure how often even the most serious of SCAM-related adverse effects occur. What we do know, however, is that under-reporting is close to 100%.[5] This leads me to conclude that the direct risks of SCAM are significantly larger than what we are currently led to believe. In this book, I will repeatedly come back to this theme and therefore not dwell on it any further at this point.

Benefits

It would be wrong to assume that all forms of SCAM are ineffective. In 2008, I published a paper[6] in which I summarised all the treatments that, according to my team's assessments, were likely to be effective [Box 4].

---

5   https://www.ncbi.nlm.nih.gov/pubmed/11285788.
6   https://www.ncbi.nlm.nih.gov/pmc/articles/PMC2249806/.

Box 4
Treatments which might generate more good than harm

Treatment	Condition	Cost	Conventional Options
Acupuncture	Nausea/vomiting	Cbc	Pme
	Osteoarthritis	Cbc	Pme
African plum (*Pygeum africanum*)	Benign prostatic hyperplasia	Moderate	Pse
Aromatherapy/massage	Cancer palliation	Cbc	Pse
Co-enzyme Q10	Hypertension	Low	Pme
Ginkgo biloba	Alzeimer's disease	Low	Pme
	Peripheral arterial disease	Low	Pme
Guar gum	Diabetes	Low	Pme
	Hypercholesterolaemia	Low	Pme
Hawthorn (*Crataegus spp.*)	Congestive heart failure	Low	Pse
Horse Chestnut (*Aesculus hippocastanum*)	Chronic venous insufficiency	Low	Pse
Hypnosis	Labour pain	Moderate	Pme
Massage	Anxiety	Cbc	Pme
Melatonin	Insomnia	Low	Pme
Music Therapy	Anxiety	Low	Pme
Padma28[b]	Peripheral arterial disease	Moderate	Pme
Phytodolor[b]	Osteoarthritis	Moderate	Pme
	Rheumatoid arthritis	Moderate	Pme
Red clover (*Trifolium pratense*)	Menopause	Moderate	Pme
Relaxation	Anxiety	Low	Pme
	Insomnia	Low	Pme
S-Adenosylmethionine	Osteoarthritis	Low	Pme
Saw palmetto (*Sereona repens*)	Benign prostatic hyperplasia	Moderate	Pse
Soy	Hypercholesterolaemia	Moderate	Pme
St John's Wort (*Hypericum perforatum*)	Depression	Moderate	Pse

This list excludes diet, vitamins, biofeedback, and preventative interventions. Cbc = can be considerable; Pme = probably more effective; Pse = probably similarly effective; [b]propriety preparation of several herbs.

Included are the treatments which were rated in 2008 as being backed up by a maximum weight of evidence demonstrating effectiveness for the condition in question.

Risk/benefit balance

I started this chapter by stressing that the value of any therapy is determined by the balance between its risks and its benefits. If the former outweigh the latter, it would be unwise to integrate the therapy in question into clinical routine.

In SCAM, the benefits are usually uncertain, small or even non-existent. In terms of risk/benefit balance, this fact is crucially important:

- If there are no benefits, the balance cannot be positive, even if the risks happen to be small.
- If the benefits are small, even relatively minor risks would produce a negative risk/benefit balance.

This means that, in SCAM, even small risks are significant determinants of the value of a therapy. It also means that few SCAMs will ever be associated with a positive risk/benefit balance. This is a theme that we will revisit regularly in the following sections of this book.

2.3. How Much of Conventional Medicine is Evidence-Based?

A major criticism of SCAM is that the evidence is often less than convincing, non-existent or negative. When discussing it with SCAM proponents, one argument is voiced regularly: 'It is unfair to insist on sound evidence for SCAM, because most of conventional medicine is also not proven.' In support of their argument, SCAM enthusiasts often cite the information from 'BMJ Clinical Evidence'.[7] It currently suggests that only a meagre 11% of conventional therapies are proven to generate benefit. An additional 24% are 'likely to be beneficial', and a whopping 50% are of 'unknown effectiveness' (the rest fall into several smaller categories such as 'unlikely to be beneficial'). Many SCAM proponents interpret these figures to mean that only 11% of what conventional clinicians do is based on sound

---

[7]   http://clinicalevidence.bmj.com/x/set/static/cms/efficacy-categorisations.html.

evidence. Therefore, they feel able to proclaim: 'the practice of conventional medicine is not evidence-based. So, why should SCAM be any better?'

The argument sounds logical. However, on closer scrutiny it turns out to be based on several misunderstandings. The above figures suggest that 35% of conventional treatments are based on compelling or at least encouraging evidence. This is far from optimal, of course, but we ought to consider that:

- The concept of evidence-based medicine is relatively new; it only started about 20 years ago.[8]
- Thousands of scientists worldwide are working tirelessly to improve the evidence base of medicine; these figures are therefore bound to improve.
- In SCAM, these percentages would surely be much worse (see previous chapter).
- The figures cited above include not just conventional therapies but also SCAMs. It is thus nonsensical to claim that the data highlight the weakness of conventional medicine. In fact, it is likely that the figures would be higher, if exclusively conventional therapies had been included in the assessment.
- The percentage figures are not a reflection of what percentages of treatments used in conventional routine are based on good evidence. Conventional clinicians would, of course, tend to select those treatments with the best evidence base, while avoiding the less well documented ones.

Several studies have investigated the last point in some detail by monitoring what proportions of interventions used by conventional clinicians in their daily practice were based on good evidence. A review of these studies[9] informs us that: *The most conclusive answer comes from a UK survey by Gill et al who retrospectively reviewed 122 consecutive general practice*

---

8   https://www.ncbi.nlm.nih.gov/pubmed/7742666.
9   https://www.ncbi.nlm.nih.gov/pmc/articles/PMC1314867/.

consultations. They found that 81% of the prescribed treatments were based on evidence and 30% were based on randomised controlled trials (RCTs). A similar study conducted in a UK university hospital outpatient department of general medicine arrived at comparable figures; 82% of the interventions were based on evidence, 53% on RCTs. Other relevant data originate from abroad. In Sweden, 84% of internal medicine interventions were based on evidence and 50% on RCTs. In Spain, these percentages were 55 and 38%, respectively. Imrie and Ramey pooled a total of 15 studies across all medical disciplines, and found that, on average, 76% of medical treatments are supported by some form of compelling evidence – the lowest was that mentioned above (55%), and the highest (97%) was achieved in anaesthesia in Britain. Collectively these data suggest that, in terms of evidence-base, general practice is much better than its reputation.

So, how much of conventional medicine is evidence-based? The answer turns out to be more complex than we may have thought, and it brings some good as well as some not so good news.

- Only a meagre 35% of conventional therapies seems to be proven or likely to generate benefit.
- However, conventional <u>practice</u> is much better than that. The best estimates indicate that 80–90% of what conventional clinicians do is based on good evidence.

The main message here is probably this: conventional medicine is not as good as we had hoped, but it is improving fast. By contrast, the evidence base for SCAM is indisputably worse, and improvement is non-existent or extremely slow.

2.4. Eminence-Based Medicine, Celebrity-Based Medicine

One striking phenomenon about SCAM is the fact that many treatments and diagnostic techniques go back to one person. This guru is revered within his field, and his ideas are elevated to a dogma (of course, in conventional medicine, this also exists, but it is far less prominent). Box 5 explains what I mean.

Box 5
SCAMs that originate from one single individual
who has attained the status of a guru in his field

- Alexander technique — F.M. Alexander
- Anthroposophical medicine — Rudolf Steiner
- Applied kinesiology — George Goodheart
- Autogenic training — H.J. Schulz
- Aromatherapy — René-Maurice Gattefossé
- Bach Flower Remedies — Edward Bach
- Bioresonance — Franz Morell
- Bowen technique — Bowen
- Craniosacral therapy — William Sutherland
- Chiropractic — D.D. Palmer
- Feldenkrais method — Moshe Feldenkrais
- German New Medicine — R.G. Hamer
- Gerson therapy — Max Gerson
- Homeopathy — Hahnemann
- Macrobiotics — George Ohsawa
- Orthomolecular medicine — Linus Pauling
- Osteopathy — Andrew Still
- Pilates — Joseph Pilates
- Reiki — Mikao Usui
- Rolfing — Ida Rolf
- Therapeutic Touch — Dolores Krieger

These men—and a few women—have all written books which serve to their followers as instruction manuals. The facts that some of these instructions originate from the pre-scientific era and most of them fly in the face of science do not seem to worry their disciples. The words of the grand master serve as a replacement for evidence. In the realm of SCAM, eminence still trumps evidence.

Those who doubt the dogma cannot be part of the cult; they are usually declared incompetent or worse and are swiftly expelled. This means that, in the eyes of the cult members, competent criticism does not exist. In this way, the cult is conveniently and permanently protected from criticism, the dogma is never endangered from within, and consequently progress is all but absent.

But how is it that some forms of eminence-based medicine can, often almost overnight, become highly popular, while others disappear just as rapidly, almost without trace. For this to happen, we need the helping hands of celebrities.

Contrary to eminence-based medicine, celebrity-based medicine[10] is a new phenomenon which was facilitated through social media. Consumers long to identify with their idols; and to achieve this aim they need to have the same clothes, cars, watches, lipstick, etc. as their idols. Consumers even want to employ the same SCAM — even if it is disproven or dangerous — and there are numerous websites where consumers can find what sort of SCAM their idols are currently embracing.

Experts are puzzled by the current popularity of SCAMs like homeopathy, for example, which has repeatedly been shown to be implausible, ineffective, costly and potentially dangerous.[11] This list of celebrities using, recommending or endorsing homeopathy goes a long way to explaining this phenomenon [Box 6].

Box 6
According to the media, homeopathy is
(or was) used by these celebrities

- Andersen, Pamela
- Becker, Boris
- Beckham, David
- Blair, Toni
- Crawford, Cindy
- Depp, Jonny
- Fonda, Jane
- Goldberg, Whoopi
- Hall, Jerry
- John, Elton
- McCartney, Paul
- Menuin, Yehudi
- Navratilova, Martina
- Newton-John, Olivia
- Turner, Tina
- Windsor, Charles
- Zeta-Jones, Catherine, and many more

---

[10] https://www.ncbi.nlm.nih.gov/pubmed/17181531.
[11] https://www.nhmrc.gov.au/guidelines-publications/cam02.

Some celebrities even have decided to make a second career in selling SCAM to the gullible public. Gwyneth Paltrow, for instance, markets all sorts of SCAMs. One of the most exotic products might be her 'jade egg'. On her website,[12] it is advertised with these words: *The strictly guarded secret of Chinese royalty in antiquity – queens and concubines used them to stay in shape for emperors – jade eggs harness the power of energy work, crystal healing, and a Kegel-like physical practice. Fans say regular use increases chi, orgasms, vaginal muscle tone, hormonal balance, and feminine energy in general. Shiva Rose has been practicing with them for about seven years, and raves about the results; we tried them, too, and were so convinced we put them into the goop shop. Jade eggs' power to cleanse and clear make them ideal for detox...*

Celebrity-based medicine relies on the innate need of humans to seek security by imitating their peers, idols and other role models. But is it a substitute for evidence? Of course not! Both eminence-based medicine and celebrity-based medicine are little more than appeals to authority,[13] a classical fallacy.

2.5. Placebo

Placebos are often employed in controlled clinical trials with the aim of differentiating the effects of the therapy *per se* and those caused by expectation and conditioning (see section 2.1). One of the first placebo-controlled studies in the history of medicine took place at the Mineral Water Hospital in Bath, UK, in 1799. It was conducted by Dr Harwarth who wanted to test an invention by Dr Elisha Perkins of Connecticut, US. Perkins had patented and popularised a device consisting of two small rods made from what he called 'secret alloys', one being the colour of brass and the other of silver. When applied to the skin and stroked downwards and outwards, these metallic 'tractors'

---

[12] http://goop.com/wellness/sexual-health/better-sex-jade-eggs-for-your-yoni/.

[13] https://en.wikipedia.org/wiki/Argument_from_authority.

relieved, according to their inventor, gout, rheumatism, headaches, epilepsy and many other disorders.

To test this device, Harwarth manufactured two wooden replicas painted in the colours of the original and he tried these 'placebos' on five rheumatic patients. Four of the patients experienced symptom relief and said they 'much benefited'. After this experiment, the real 'tractors' were used in the same way. The results were identical, 'distinctly proving to what a surprising degree mere fancy deceives the patient'.

This early attempt to differentiate between the specific and the non-specific effect of a medical treatment tells us a great deal about placebos [Box 7]. Clinicians, past and present, conventional or alternative, cannot normally differentiate between placebo effects and specific effects of their treatments, unless they make a conscious and often laborious effort of the kind Harwarth undertook in 1799. They may read about placebos and understand the concept, but they will rarely attribute any clinical improvement to the placebo effect. Therefore, they tend to conclude that the placebo effect plays no role in their practice because they only use effective treatments.

Yet, in clinical practice, there is only one situation where placebo effects might be recognised with some degree of certainty, and it hardly ever occurs. It is when a practitioner intentionally administers an inert treatment to a patient. Today, few healthcare practitioners will ever do such a thing; most feel that this would be dishonest. Clinicians therefore never consciously see pure placebo effects. Instead, they witness clinical outcomes which normally rely on a complex mix of the specific effects of the prescribed treatment and non-specific effects (e.g. placebo effect, regression towards the mean, natural history of the disease) which we often, but somewhat incorrectly, call 'placebo'. Virtually any treatment administered to patients would result in such a mixture of specific and non-specific effects. The exact composition of the mix will vary depending on the therapy, the therapist, the interaction between them, and many other variables.

The remarkable phenomenon that non-specific effects are usually mistaken for specific effects of treatments is, I am sure, a prime reason for the survival of ineffective and even hazardous treatments. Blood-letting and purging — treatments which killed many more patients than they ever helped — are examples from the past; and some currently popular forms of SCAMs, e.g. homeopathy, crystal or spiritual healing, are examples from the present.

Some people argue that treatments like homeopathy are acceptable, even if they are pure placebos. After all, they say, it helps many patients regardless of the mechanism of action. This assumption neglects the fact that the use of placebos in routine healthcare is highly problematic. In conditions for which effective curative or symptomatic treatments exist, it might delay or prevent access to such therapies. Using placebos in this way would be ethically and legally wrong and a disservice to the patient.

Yet, whenever a form of SCAM has been shown to be ineffective, i.e. not superior to placebo, its proponents claim that it nevertheless helps many patients via a placebo effect. This argument suggests that the therapy has no specific effect but leads to a substantial non-specific (placebo) response which, after all, benefits suffering patients. Thus, a scientist testing it against placebo is likely to call it 'ineffective', while many SCAM practitioners and their patients might value it as 'effective'.

Differentiating between specific and non-specific therapeutic effects is not just a question of terminology, even though for the patient it may look like splitting hairs — all the patient wants is to get better. For improving healthcare and for the benefit of tomorrow's patients, the distinction matters greatly and unquestionably.

- If a placebo carries significant risks, as some SCAMs clearly do, we must ask ourselves whether the placebo response might not be achieved with a less risky treatment.

- If it is expensive, we should look for a cheaper treatment.
- If it means that patients are led to believe in the paranormal or absurd (e.g. spiritual healing), we ought to find a more rational therapy.

The most crucial point, however, is that even effective treatments invariably come with the 'free bonus' of non-specific effects. All the non-specific effects are, of course, operative regardless of whether a patient takes an active medicine or a sugar pill. Patients' needs are undoubtedly served best if both specific and non-specific effects are employed for their benefit. It follows that a treatment which relies on nothing more than placebo effects is not usually an acceptable therapy. Or, to put it even more bluntly, the placebo effect alone is no justification for using medical interventions such as SCAM.

Further important reasons for differentiating transparently between specific and non-specific therapeutic effects are scientific honesty and progress. Honesty is a value that cannot be rated highly enough. Progress is equally important. If we are simply content with the view that all is fine 'as long as it helps patients', without trying to define the exact causes of clinical improvement, we are unlikely to advance in our endeavour to create a better healthcare for tomorrow.

BOX 7
Some intriguing facts about placebo

- The first mention of 'placebo' in an English medical dictionary was in 1785.
- Placebo was not mentioned in a French medical dictionary until 1958.
- Placebo surgery, surgical incisions under anaesthesia without the actual operation, has repeatedly been shown to alleviate symptoms effectively.
- Placebos seem to act via the same mechanisms as the active drug would. For instance, placebo painkillers activate the same areas of the brain as the real painkiller would.
- More invasive placebos (e.g. saline injections) tend to generate greater placebo effects than placebo pills.
- A dose–response relationship has been noted: the size of the placebo effect increases if the placebo is given more frequently.
- Placebos can also cause unwanted effects, called nocebo effects.
- European studies tend to show larger placebo effects than American investigations.

2.6. Ethical Issues in Scam

Medical ethics provides a system of moral principles that apply to healthcare. Its principal values are:

- Autonomy — respecting the rights of patients,
- Beneficence — doing good,
- and non-maleficence — doing no harm.

Medical ethics is central to any type of healthcare — and this includes, of course, SCAM. Many of the issues discussed in this book are at their core issues of medical ethics, and the often-sceptical stance of conventional doctors towards SCAM has its roots in concerns about the numerous violations of ethical standards in this area.

The American Medical Association (AMA) recently published a document entitled 'The Modernized AMA *Code of Medical Ethics*'.[14] The following 9 points are from this code; in brackets are my own comments pertaining specifically to SCAM. Most of the issues mentioned here merely in passing will be discussed in more detail elsewhere in this book.

1. A physician shall be dedicated to providing competent medical care, with compassion and respect for human dignity and rights. [Most SCAM practitioners use unproven treatments of one type or another; it seems doubtful whether administering unproven therapies can qualify as 'competent medical care'.]
2. A physician shall uphold the standards of professionalism, be honest in all professional interactions, and strive to report physicians deficient in character or competence, or engaging in fraud or deception, to appropriate entities. [Treating patients with unproven therapies is arguably unprofessional, dishonest and deceptive, particularly in the absence of fully informed consent (see below).]

---

[14]   http://jamanetwork.com/journals/jama/article-abstract/2534495.

3. A physician shall respect the law and also recognise a responsibility to seek changes in those requirements which are contrary to the best interests of the patient. [Treatment with unproven therapies, while omitting proven interventions, cannot be in the best interest of the patient.]

4. A physician shall respect the rights of patients, colleagues and other health professionals, and shall safeguard patient confidences and privacy within the constraints of the law. [The right of patients includes full informed consent which is a rarity in SCAM (see below).]

5. A physician shall continue to study, apply and advance scientific knowledge, maintain a commitment to medical education, make relevant information available to patients, colleagues and the public, obtain consultation, and use the talents of other health professionals when indicated. [SCAM is frequently out of line with or even opposed to scientific and medical knowledge.]

6. A physician shall, in the provision of appropriate patient care, except in emergencies, be free to choose whom to serve, with whom to associate, and the environment in which to provide medical care.

7. A physician shall recognise a responsibility to participate in activities contributing to the improvement of the community and the betterment of public health. [Some activities of some SCAM practitioners are directly opposed to public health, for example the advice of many homeopaths, chiropractors, naturopaths and anthroposophic physicians against immunising children.[15, 16, 17]]

---

15 https://www.ncbi.nlm.nih.gov/pubmed/11587822.
16 https://www.ncbi.nlm.nih.gov/pubmed/12559777.
17 https://www.ncbi.nlm.nih.gov/pubmed/21102363.

8. A physician shall, while caring for a patient, regard responsibility to the patient as paramount. [It seems doubtful whether this is possible when using unproven therapies.]

9. A physician shall support access to medical care for all people. [Some SCAM practitioners advise their patients against accessing conventional healthcare such as vaccinations (see above).]

These comments go some way towards explaining why medical ethics is a problem for SCAM providers: if ethical principles were truly applied in SCAM, much of today's SCAM practice would have to change radically or stop altogether.

In the following subsections, I will focus on just two specific ethical issues that are, in my view, particularly pertinent to SCAM: informed consent and conflicts of interest (other ethical issues are discussed elsewhere in this book; see for instance section 6.5).

Informed consent

Before starting treatment or initiating a diagnostic procedure, all healthcare professionals — including, of course, SCAM practitioners — must obtain informed consent. This is by no means optional but an ethical and legal imperative. Informed consent should usually include full information on:

- the diagnosis
- the natural history of the condition
- the most effective treatment options available for the condition
- the proposed therapy
- its effectiveness
- its risks
- its cost
- a rough treatment plan

Only when this information has been transmitted to and understood by the patient can informed consent be considered complete. But is such complete consent even possible in the realm of SCAM? I will use two fictional but nevertheless realistic scenarios to explore this question.

SCENARIO 1

A patient with fatigue and headaches consults a Reiki healer. The Reiki master asks a few questions about the patient's history and symptoms and proceeds to apply Reiki. He has no means of obtaining informed consent because:

- he is not qualified to make a reasonable diagnosis,
- he knows little about the natural history of the patient's condition,
- he is ignorant of the most effective treatment options conventional medicine has to offer for the patient's condition,
- he is convinced that Reiki works and unaware of the evidence which is largely negative.

SCENARIO 2

The same patient with fatigue and headaches consults a chiropractor. The chiropractor takes a history, conducts a physical examination, tells the patient that her headaches are due to spinal misalignments which he suggests treating with spinal manipulations, and proceeds to apply his treatments. The chiropractor has no means of obtaining informed consent because:

- he has insufficient knowledge of conventional therapeutic options,
- he is biased as to the effectiveness of spinal manipulations,
- he believes that they are virtually risk-free,
- he has an overt conflict of interest (see below).

These scenarios were chosen to explain why, in SCAM, informed consent might often be unachievable. Put simply, informed consent requires knowledge that SCAM providers rarely possess. Moreover, it requires a lack of financial interest such that the clinician is not in danger of losing out on some income, in case he advises his patient not to receive treatment from him. Finally, informed consent requires information about the treatment, including explanations as to how it works. For most SCAMs, this information does not exist and therefore cannot be provided.

These considerations highlight profound differences between SCAM and conventional medicine relating to the competence of the clinicians involved. At medical school, doctors-to-be learn myriad necessary facts enabling them to adequately deal with the obligatory elements of informed consent. By contrast, most SCAM practitioners have gone through a type of training—if they have any formal training at all—which has not provided them with this knowledge.

There is little research to tell us how often SCAM practitioners try employing informed consent in their daily routine. One laudable exception is a survey of 200 UK chiropractors which indicated that only 45% always discuss the risks with patients in need of cervical manipulation.[18] A second survey showed that the US situation is similar. The authors concluded that *'a patient's autonomy and right to self-determination may be compromised when seeking chiropractic care'*.[19] Considering that, in these surveys, the truthfulness of the responses by the participating chiropractors could not be verified, it seems safe to assume that reality might even be worse than these articles suggest.

In research, informed consent is at least as important as it is in clinical practice. Before entering patients into a clinical trial, it is mandatory to obtain their informed consent along the lines explained above. In SCAM research, this aspect seems often to get neglected. In a 2004 survey of published SCAM articles, we found that 52% of them failed to report that the investigators had obtained informed consent from their patients.[20]

---

[18]   https://www.ncbi.nlm.nih.gov/pubmed/20977721.
[19]   https://www.ncbi.nlm.nih.gov/pubmed/17693332.
[20]   https://www.ncbi.nlm.nih.gov/pubmed/15379147.

In the interest of honesty, I should admit that I was once accused of conducting research without informed consent. In my memoir, I recount the full story:

In 2002, at the time of the MMR (measles, mumps, and rubella vaccine) scare promoted by Andrew Wakefield's now discredited 'research', we decided to broaden our initial pilot-study to the national level. In order to accomplish this, we had obtained the email addresses of a sizeable number of UK chiropractors and homeopaths, and sent a request to these practitioners. In it, a fictional mother, concerned about the conflicting press reports regarding the safety of the MMR vaccine, asked for advice on MMR vaccination for her one-year-old child. After the replies had come in, we wrote to each respondent again and explained that the query had not been genuine but was, in fact, part of a research project. At the same time, we offered all participants the chance to withdraw their answers. The study had, of course, been approved in advance by our local ethics committee, and debriefing the respondents in this way was part of the approved protocol.

In total, we managed to contact 168 homeopaths, of whom 72 per cent responded, and 26 per cent withdrew their answers after the debriefing. We also contacted 63 chiropractors, of whom 44 per cent responded initially and 27 per cent later withdrew their responses. Our analyses showed that very few homeopaths and only a quarter of the chiropractors would advise their patients in favour of the MMR vaccination. Almost half of the homeopaths and nearly a fifth of the chiropractors would recommend against immunising.

What happened next is amazing and perhaps even unprecedented in the recent history of medical research. This seemingly innocent and insignificant research project almost cost me my job. After receiving the debriefing email, several homeopaths complained to my university peers and to our ethics committee, claiming the research was unethical because it had been conducted on non-consenting human research subjects (the homeopaths and chiropractors) who had been misled about the nature of the inquiry. In view of these complaints, our ethics committee got cold feet and took the most remarkable step of withdrawing their previous approval; not only that, they forbade us to use the results in any way.

However, at this stage of the project, I had already submitted our findings as a short report for publication in the *British Medical Journal*, and I flatly refused to comply with those ridiculous demands. The article was thus published only days after this storm had started blowing.

My Exeter peers were not amused by my disobedience, decided to conduct an official investigation and ordered me to attend several interrogatory sessions. For several weeks, I thought they might find me guilty of conducting unethical research and condemn my actions which, in the worst-case scenario, could have meant disciplinary action against me. Even the mildest reprimand would have been devastating to the credibility of my research team as a whole. The homeopaths who had filed the complaint were only waiting to use such news to discredit me once and for all. Fortunately, after several highly unpleasant exchanges, I managed to convince my peers that, considering the lively public and medical debate about the risks or benefits of the MMR vaccination, a swift publication of these findings had been in the public's best interest. Eventually, it was decided that no disciplinary action, not even a reprimand, was called for.

I felt strongly then—and I still do today—that our research was not in the least unethical. In order to discover the extent and the effects of irresponsible behaviour, researchers, like police, sometimes have no choice but to conduct undercover investigations of this nature; and, whenever necessary, I continued doing so.

Conflicts of interest

When researchers publish a paper, they must disclose all conflicts of interest. The aim of this exercise is to be as transparent as possible. The questionnaires that authors complete prior to publication of their article usually focus on financial issues. For instance, one must disclose any sponsorship, fees, travel support or shares that one might own in a company. In conventional medicine, these matters are deemed to be the most important sources for potential conflicts of interest. In SCAM, financial issues are generally thought to be far less critical because SCAM is usually seen as an area that involves little money. Perhaps this is the reason why few SCAM journals (see section 4.10) insist on declarations of conflicts of interests and few authors disclose them.[21]

One example must stand for many that I personally witnessed. The senior author of a 2008 paper[22] reporting an observational study of homeopathy chose to publish it under the UK address of 'International Institute for Integrated Medicine'. He seemed to have forgotten that, at the time, he also was employed as a consultant for a homeopathic company. As this firm also happened to be the manufacturer of the homeopathic remedy used for the study, this omission is a little more than embarrassing, in my view.

In my experience, conflicts of interest are at least as prevalent and powerful in SCAM as in other areas of healthcare. Quasi-evangelic convictions abound in SACM, and it is obvious that they can amount to significant conflicts of interest. This is not just true for research but also for clinical practice. During their training, SCAM practitioners learn many things which are unproven, have no basis in fact, or are just plainly wrong. For example:

---

[21] https://www.ncbi.nlm.nih.gov/pubmed/15379147.
[22] https://www.ncbi.nlm.nih.gov/pubmed/?term=scneider+c%2C+van+has elen+r.

- chiropractors learn the assumptions of D.D. Palmer are correct;
- homeopaths learn the assumptions of S. Hahnemann are correct;
- osteopaths learn the assumptions of A. Still are correct;
- flower therapists learn the assumptions of doctor E. Bach are correct;
- anthroposophical physicians learn the assumptions of R. Steiner are correct.

This 'education' creates a belief system which is usually adhered to regardless of the scientific evidence and which tends to be defended at all cost. Students of chiropractic, for example, develop an increasingly strong opinion against vaccinations, which is due to the type of information they receive at the chiropractic college (D.D. Palmer was an outspoken opponent of immunisation).[23] Creeds can easily represent an even more powerful conflict of interest than financial matters.

In the daily routine of SCAM practice, this belief is indivisibly intertwined with existential issues. There may not be vast amounts of money at stake, but SCAM practitioners' livelihoods are perceived to be at risk nevertheless. If an acupuncturist, for instance, argues in favour of his therapy, he is consciously or subconsciously trying to protect his income.

Some might argue that, in conventional medicine, things are just as bad or even worse. But there is one stark difference. If we take away one specific therapy from doctors—because it turns out to be useless or unsafe, for instance—they will not lose out financially because they are able to use another treatment instead. If, by contrast, we take the acupuncture needle away from an acupuncturist, we have deprived him of his livelihood. Therefore, conflicts of interest in SCAM tend to be very acute, powerful and personal. Consequently, SCAM

---

23   http://www.tihcij.com/Articles/Anti-Vaccination-Attitudes-within-the-Chiropractic-Profession-Implications-for-Public-Health-Ethics.aspx?id= 0000377.

practitioners are often incapable or unwilling to look upon any type of critical assessment of their area as anything other than a threat to their income, their beliefs, their status, their training or their person.

But what about my very own conflicts of interest?

This is, of course, a fair question, not least because the reader of this book has a right to know how impartial I am. Many SCAM proponents seem to be convinced that, back in 1993, when I accepted the job as Professor of Complementary Medicine at the University of Exeter, I had a hidden agenda. They claim that I was determined — or perhaps even paid — to show that all SCAM is hocus-pocus.

The truth is that, if anything, I was on the side of SCAM — and, what is more, I can even prove it! Using the example of homeopathy, I have dedicated an entire paper[24] to providing evidence demonstrating that I was not closed-minded or out to ditch homeopathy (or any other form of SCAM for that matter).

Unfortunately, rational arguments never convince fanatics. One of my most determined critics even filed an official 'freedom of information request' with my University to obtain the details about the origins of my research funding. The answer revealed that the core funds came from 'The Laing Foundation', which endowed Exeter University with £1.5 million. This was done with the understanding that Exeter would raise the same amount again (which they never did). In addition, I managed to receive financial support for multiple research fellowships from various sources; for instance, manufacturers of herbal medicines, 'Boots the Chemist', and the Pilkington Family Trust. Further contributors were the roughly 30 visiting scientists from abroad who came on their own money simply because they wanted to learn from and with us. We also devised numerous ways to generate our own research funds. For instance, we started an annual conference for SCAM researchers which ran for 14 years and made a tidy profit each

---

[24] https://www.ncbi.nlm.nih.gov/pubmed/19832813.

year. Furthermore, we published several books which generated some revenue. Finally, we received research funding for specific projects—for instance, from The Prince Of Wales' Foundation for Integrated Health, a Japanese organisation supporting Johrei Healing, The Wellcome Trust, the NHS, as well as several herbal and homeopathic manufacturers.

And today? Well, today I live off my pension and my savings. I am not on the payroll of anyone, and nobody (except the publisher) is paying me for writing this book.

So, do I have a conflict of interest?

Not in the sense some of my opponents claim. But I do have a different and perhaps more important type of conflict. I strongly believe that:

- evidence is a prerequisite for progress in healthcare,
- evidence must be established by rigorous research,
- we should not tolerate double standards in healthcare,
- patients deserve to be treated with the best available treatments,
- making therapeutic claims that are not supported by sound evidence is wrong.

These convictions seem to make me biased in the eyes of some SCAM practitioners. For example, several acupuncturists[25] seem to think that I have always been against acupuncture for the sake of being against acupuncture. Yet, I have published many articles that concluded positively. One of our meta-analyses,[26] for instance, concluded: *Acupuncture effectively relieves chronic low back pain.* (This, of course, was years ago when the evidence was, in fact, positive; today, this has changed.)

And what about the conflicts of interest of my detractors? What about the acupuncturists mentioned above, for example?

---

[25] http://edzardernst.com/2016/03/nice-no-longer-recommends-acupuncture-chiropractic-or-osteopathy-for-low-back-pain/.

[26] https://www.ncbi.nlm.nih.gov/pubmed/?term=ernst%2C+manheimer%2C+acupuncture%2C+back+pain.

- They earn their money with acupuncture.
- They have invested in their acupuncture training.
- They have invested in practice equipment, etc.
- And all of them have strong beliefs about acupuncture.

The message that seems to emerge from all this is simple, albeit somewhat disturbing: those SCAM proponents who accuse their critics of having significant conflicts of interest are usually the only ones who are burdened with conflicts of interest.

Chapter 3

Common Problems in SCAM

*I have yet to see any problem, however complicated, which,
when you looked at it in the right way, did not become still
more complicated. — Poul Anderson*

3.1. The Root Cause and the Panacea

In discussions with SCAM practitioners about the 'pros and
cons' of their therapies, it is almost inevitable that, sooner or
later, someone claims '**WE** TREAT THE ROOT CAUSES OF
DISEASE!!!'. The statement is regularly pronounced with deep
conviction, and it seems clear that the practitioners fully and
wholeheartedly believe it. How could it be otherwise?

- The message is simple and attractive.
- It is being taught in virtually all SCAM schools, semi-
  nars, books, etc.
- It is good for business.

But, unfortunately, the message is not correct. It is misleading
in that it implies that conventional clinicians do not care about
the 'root causes of disease'. The truth is that, whenever possible, conventional doctors try to identify the cause of any symptom or disease and subsequently treat it. A simple example is a
patient with fever and breathing problems; his doctor diagnoses bacterial pneumonia and treats the root cause of the
disease with antibiotics.

But the above claim, 'WE TREAT THE ROOT CAUSES OF DISEASE', is not just misleading, it also is demonstrably wrong. It is based on SCAM practitioners' understanding of aetiology [Box 8].

Box 8
The root causes of disease as seen
by various SCAM practitioners

- If a traditional acupuncturist is convinced that all disease is the expression of an imbalance of yin and yang, and that needling acu-puncture points will re-balance these vital energies, thus restoring health, he must automatically assume that he is treating the **root causes** of any condition.
- If a chiropractor believes in D.D. Palmer's gospel that all diseases are due to 'subluxations' of the spine, it must seem logical to him that spinal 'adjustment' is synonymous with treating the **root cause** of whatever complaint his patient is suffering from.
- If a Bowen therapist is convinced that his treatment re-balances the whole person, he is bound to be sure that he tackles the **root causes** of any health problem.
- If an energy healer believes that a patient's complaints are due to his vital energy failing, and that the healer's ability to channel energy into his body will restore the deficit, he will be convinced that he is addressing the **root causes** of all or most diseases.
- If a homeopath has been taught that the **root cause** of all health prob-lems lies in a lack of vital energy which must be restored with a carefully chosen homeopathic remedy, he must assume he can treat any human condition.

But let us pretend for a minute that SCAM practitioners are correct in believing that their interventions are therapies directed against the cause of a disease. Successful treatment of any root cause means that the therapy in question heals the problem at hand. If we eliminate the cause of a disease, we would expect the disease to disappear for good.

So, are there diseases that can be cured by SCAM? I have never been able to identify a single one. Even those SCAMs that are demonstrably effective (see section 2.2) are not causal treatments, but they are symptomatic by nature. A good example is perhaps St John's Wort, the herbal remedy that has been shown to be an effective treatment for mild to moderate depression.[1] Yes, it is effective, but only in a symptomatic fashion. It alleviates the symptoms of depression, but not its cause. Once a depressed patient stops taking this herbal remedy, her depression is likely to return.

The claim of being able to tackle the root causes of disease is, of course, closely related to SCAM practitioners' often-voiced claim that their specific type of SCAM is a panacea, a 'cure-all'. Based on the naïve conviction that all conditions are due to one single cause and that this root cause can be tackled by their therapy, many SCAM practitioners believe that they are able to treat all or most conditions [Box 9].

Box 9
SCAMs are often promoted as cure-alls

- A homeopath believes that all diseases are due to the patient's impeded vital force; thus, all conditions would respond to its activation via homeopathy.
- A traditional acupuncturist believes that all diseases are due to an imbalance of yin and yang; thus, all conditions would respond to re-balancing them with acupuncture.
- A chiropractor believes that all diseases are due to subluxations; thus, all conditions would respond to adjusting them with spinal manipulations.
- An energy healer believes that all diseases are due to blockages of our vital energy; thus, all conditions would respond to de-blocking them via energy healing.

Not only do many SCAM practitioners believe that their SCAM is a panacea, but they bombard the public with this message in articles, books, lectures, etc., thereby reinforcing and popularising this myth. There are virtually thousands of examples for this, but here two will have to suffice.

The first originates from a manufacturer of natural medicines and beauty products who published an article entitled 'An Introduction to Homeopathy'.[2] In it, we find the following revealing statement: *Homeopathy can be used to treat the same wide range of illness as conventional medicine, and may even prove*

---

[1]   https://www.ncbi.nlm.nih.gov/pubmed/28083422.
[2]   https://www.weleda.co.uk/homeopathy?utm_medium=email&utm_source=apsis-anp-3.

successful when all other forms of treatment have failed. Its meaning could not be clearer: homeopathy is a panacea.

Should we believe this claim? I suggest, rather, we believe any of the official verdicts issued by the organisations listed below:[3]

> The principles of homeopathy contradict known chemical, physical and biological laws and persuasive scientific trials proving its effectiveness are not available. (Russian Academy of Sciences, Russia)

> Homeopathy should not be used to treat health conditions that are chronic, serious, or could become serious. People who choose homeopathy may put their health at risk if they reject or delay treatments for which there is good evidence for safety and effectiveness. (National Health and Medical Research Council, Australia)

> These products are not supported by scientific evidence. (Health Canada, Canada)

> Homeopathic remedies don't meet the criteria of evidence based medicine. (Hungarian Academy of Sciences, Hungary)

> The incorporation of anthroposophical and homeopathic products in the Swedish directive on medicinal products would run counter to several of the fundamental principles regarding medicinal products and evidence-based medicine. (Swedish Academy of Sciences, Sweden)

> We recommend parents and caregivers not give homeopathic teething tablets and gels to children and seek advice from their health care professional for safe alternatives. (Food and Drug Administration, USA)

---

[3]   http://edzardernst.com/2017/04/official-verdicts-on-homeopathy/.

There is little evidence to support homeopathy as an effective treatment for any specific condition. (National Centre for Complementary and Integrative Health, USA)

There is no good-quality evidence that homeopathy is effective as a treatment for any health condition. (National Health Service, UK)

Homeopathic remedies perform no better than placebos, and that the principles on which homeopathy is based are 'scientifically implausible'. (House of Commons Science and Technology Committee, UK)

The second example relates to pranic healing. In case you are not sure what this SCAM is, the following excerpt explains:[4]

Pranic Healing is a form of ancient energy medicine, which utilizes the inherent energy Prana (life force or energy) to balance, and promote the body's energy and its processes. Prana is a Sanskrit word which actually means, the vital force that keeps us alive and healthy... Following health issues can be successfully treated with Pranic healing:
• Sleeping illness (lack of sleep)
• Mental illnesses including depression, anxiety etc.
• Stress
• Sprains and strains
• Body aches like neck pain, muscle pain, back pain etc.
• A recent trauma and related inflammation
• Improve psycho-physical aspects in athletes
• Improve memory
• Enhance energy level
• Treat headache
• Fight ulcers (intestinal)
• Heal respiratory illnesses, including sinusitis and asthma
• Skin diseases, including eczema
• Improves overall immunity
• Treat the various causes of infertility

---

4   http://www.desimd.com/alternative-medicine/ayurveda/pranic-healing.

- Aesthetic treatments such as Pranic face lift, bust lift, hip and tummy tuck etc.

Should we believe these therapeutic claims made for pranic healing? Not without evidence, I suggest. So, where is the evidence? The largest electronic database in healthcare, Medline, lists just 4 articles on pranic healing.

- The first paper[5] is entirely evidence-free, but we do learn the following: *When Pranic healing is applied the molecular structure of liquid and dense states of matter can be altered significantly to create positive outcomes, as revealed through research.*
- The second paper[6] is not actually on pranic healing and contains no relevant information about it.
- The third paper[7] is an oddly promotional essay for nurses and fails to include anything resembling evidence.
- And the fourth paper[8] is yet another evidence-free, promotional article.

It would be wonderful if we had a treatment that was a 'cure-all'. However, the truth is a far cry from the panacea myth: no SCAM tackles the root causes of disease, and no SCAM (or conventional therapy) can cure all diseases. In fact, I am not aware of a single SCAM that can cure a single disease.

3.2. Fear-Mongering

For more than two decades, I have consistently been warning about the risks of SCAM, and I must have published well over 100 papers on this very issue. One of my first articles[9] on safety concerns was published in 1995 and focused on the risks of acupuncture. Here is it's a short extract:

---

5   https://www.ncbi.nlm.nih.gov/pubmed/19175256.
6   https://www.ncbi.nlm.nih.gov/pubmed/15040779.
7   https://www.ncbi.nlm.nih.gov/pubmed/12889412.
8   https://www.ncbi.nlm.nih.gov/pubmed/12056313.
9   https://www.ncbi.nlm.nih.gov/pubmed/23511615.

The repeated and/or inappropriate use of an acupuncture needle carries the risk of infections. Amongst others, AIDS and hepatitis have been transmitted. Acupuncture needles may also traumatise tissues and organs. Pneumothorax is the most frequent complication caused in this way. Finally, needles may break and fragments can be dislodged into distant organs. A serious and more general concern related to the safety of acupuncture is the competence of the therapist, whether or not medically qualified. The 'philosophy' of acupuncture is not in line with orthodox diagnostic skills; therefore, acupuncturists can be dangerously unconcerned with diagnostic categories. Thus, indirect risks might add significantly to the direct risks of acupuncture.

My reason for continuing to write about the potential harms of SCAM (see also section 2.2) is neither axe-grinding nor fear-mongering, but an ethical and moral duty: I feel obliged to alert the public to the fact that SCAM may not be as harmless as it is usually advertised to be. For me, there is no subject in medicine that is more important than the safety of patients, and consumers.

Yet, proponents of SCAM often accuse me of being an alarmist fear-monger. In my view, nothing could be further from the truth, and I often cannot fail to notice that those who accuse me are the ones guilty of the deed. So, is it true, are SCAM practitioners fear-mongers? Surely not all of them, but some clearly are.

Perhaps the most obvious way SCAM practitioners instil fear into people is to tell them that they are affected by a disease or condition they do not have.

- A chiropractor will tell you that you have a subluxation in your spine.
- A naturopath would inform you that your body is full of toxins.
- An acupuncturist will tell you that your chi is blocked.
- A homeopath might warn you that your vital force is failing.

These diagnoses have one thing in common: they do not exist. They are figments of the therapist's imagination. Yet SCAM providers would insist that these mystical abnormalities need to be corrected, and—surprise, surprise—that the very therapy in which they specialise happens to be just the ticket for that purpose.

- The chiropractor will tell you that a simple spinal adjustment will solve the problem.
- The naturopath will inform you that his detox treatments will eliminate the toxins.
- The acupuncturist will convince you that his needles will de-block your chi.
- The homeopath will persuade you that he can find the exact remedy to revive your vital force.

Of course, imagined diagnoses and subsequent treatments invariably result in a bill which, in turn, improves the cash-flow of the therapist.

But, often, it is not even necessary for a SCAM practitioner to completely invent a diagnosis. Patients usually consult a therapist with some sort of symptom—frequently with what one might call a medical triviality that does not need any treatment at all, but can be dealt with differently, for instance, by issuing some lifestyle advice, or just simple reassurance that nothing major is amiss. But for the fear-monger, this is not enough. He feels the need to administer his therapy, and for that purpose he needs to medicalise trivialities:

- A low mood thus becomes a clinical depression.
- A sore back is turned into a nasty lumbago.
- A tummy upset morphs into a dangerous gastritis.
- Abdominal unrest is diagnosed to be a leaky gut syndrome.
- A mere aversion turns into a food intolerance, etc., etc.

The principle is simple enough: fear is instilled into the patient, and SCAM must be administered—if at all possible in the form of a lengthy series of treatments. This, of course, generates significant benefit—not therapeutic, but financial; and not for the patient, but for the therapist.

But what if the patient is wiser than expected? She might be so fearful after learning of her condition that she decides to see a real doctor. For the SCAM therapist, that would mean a loss of income, a development which, of course, must be avoided. To achieve this aim, conventional healthcare professionals must be demonised; and for that aim, no tale is too tall:

- They are not treating the root cause of the problem (see previous section).
- They are in the pocket of Big Pharma.
- They prescribe medicines with terrible side effects.
- They have no idea about holism (see next section).
- They never have enough time to listen, etc., etc.

Some of these criticisms are, of course, not entirely incorrect (for instance, many conventional medicines do have serious side effects; however, we need to consider their risk/benefit balance for defining their true value, see section 2.2). But that is hardly the point here; the point is to scare the patient off conventional medicine. Only a person who is convinced that the 'medical mafia' is out to get her will prove to be a loyal customer of SCAM.

And a loyal customer is someone who comes not just once or twice but regularly, ideally from 'cradle to grave'. The way to achieve this ultimate stimulus of the practitioner's cash flow is to convince the patient that she needs regular treatments, even during times when she feels perfectly fine. The magic word here is PREVENTION! Chiropractors, for instance, promote what they call 'maintenance care', i.e. the regular treatment of healthy individuals to keep their spines subluxation-free. (It goes almost without saying that maintenance care has not been shown to be effective in preventing anything other than poverty of chiropractors.[10])

---

[10]   https://www.ncbi.nlm.nih.gov/pubmed/19465044.

The strategy requires two little untruths, but that must be forgivable considering the noble cause of boosting the income of the SCAM practitioner:

1. Conventional doctors do not care about prevention.
2. The SCAM in question is an effective preventative.

The first statement is, of course, plainly wrong. Everything we know today about effective disease prevention originated from conventional medicine and science; nothing came from the realm of SCAM. (Intriguingly, the most efficacious preventative measure of all time, immunisation, is frequently disregarded or defamed by SCAM practitioners.[11]) The second statement is an equally obvious untruth. I am not aware of any SCAM that can effectively prevent any disease, and the many practitioners who I have asked could not name one either.

What follows from all this is, as depressing as it is, I think, undeniable:

- Some SCAM practitioners regularly try to instil fear into consumers.
- A range of strategies are commonly being used for this purpose.
- The aim of this fear-mongering is to maximise the SCAM therapists' income.

3.3. Holism

Our local bakery is an example of true holism. The first thing that strikes me when I enter its premises is the irresistible smell. Customers' well-being hits the ceiling, and the local aroma-therapists are out of business. The intense stimulation of the olfactory system relaxes everyone's mind; it lulls me into an autohypnotic state as I wait to be served. 'You're looking well today', says the baker's wife with a smile. Her diagnosis is spot on; her holistic therapy has already cured all my ills. Her

---

[11] http://pediatrics.aappublications.org/content/early/2016/09/30/peds.2015-4664.

wholewheat cheese scones are unbeatable so I order three — one for the road and two for tea at home. Prices have gone up a bit, but, as with all holistic therapies, the more you pay the more it's worth. 'Here you are', she says, handing me my scones. As I pay, our hands touch and I briefly experience the transfer of vital energy characteristic of all touch therapies. 'Take care now, and God bless.' As I walk home, I contemplate this extraordinary experience — holistically embracing body, mind, spirit and soul.

I know, holism is a serious subject, and I should not joke about it. But it is also a much-abused issue, particularly in SCAM.

Holism is an essential characteristic of all good medicine; without it, healthcare is defective:

> It is a common misconception that holistic medicine is just 'alternative' or 'complementary' medicine. Clinical holistic medicine actually dates as far back as Hippocrates. An holistic approach to patient care was also suggested by Percival in his book — the first textbook of medical ethics — first published in 1803. Percival stated: 'The feeling and emotions of the patients require to be known and to be attended to, no less than the symptoms of their diseases.' More recently, John Macleod in his book 'Clinical Examination', first published in 1964, also commented that 'we should aim to be holistic in our care'. Also, the seminal work by Michael Balint, 'The Doctor, the Patient and his Illness', first published in 1957, represents an important landmark in seeing the patient as a whole rather than as isolated pathology... An holistic approach is good practice and has been strongly advocated by the Royal College of General Practitioners for many years.[12]

Proponents of SCAM, however, tend to see this differently. They have jumped on the 'holistic band-wagon' and seem to think that they now own it: they imply that they are the only

---

[12]　https://patient.info/doctor/holistic-medicine.

clinicians who practise holistically. This, of course, has the added benefit of putting people off conventional medicine because it is characterised as non-holistic.

Yet, the claim that all SCAM is holistic usually turns out to be false: much of SCAM is exactly the opposite of holistic. Take, for instance, the example of acupuncture for neck pain (I could have used almost any other SCAM and any other human complaint, condition or disease). A recent study[13] found that adding acupuncture to usual care yields a slightly better outcome than usual care alone. This is hardly surprising; adding a good cup of tea or a compassionate chat to usual care might have had a similar effect. Acupuncturists, however, claim that their holistic approach is successful. But how holistic is acupuncture?

When seeing a new patient, a 'Western' acupuncturist would normally enquire what is wrong with the patient; in the case of neck pain, he would probably ask several further questions about the history of the condition, when the pain occurs, what aggravates it, etc. Then he might conduct a physical examination of his patient. Eventually, he would get out his needles and start the treatment.

A 'traditional' acupuncturist, i.e. one who adheres to the principles of Traditional Chinese Medicine, would ask similar questions, feel the pulse, look at the tongue and make a diagnosis in terms of yin and yang imbalance or blocked chi. Eventually, he too would get out his needles and start the treatment.

In either of these instances, I fail to see how the approach can be characterised as holistic. In fact, most SCAM practitioners tend to be the very opposite of holistic. Holistic means that the patient is understood as a whole person — body, mind and spirit. Our neck pain patient might have physical problems such as muscular tension; the acupuncturists might well have realised this and placed their needles accordingly. But neck

---

[13] http://annals.org/aim/article/2467961/alexander-technique-lessons-acupuncture-sessions-persons-chronic-neck-pain-randomized.

pain, like most other symptoms, often has several other dimensions:

- there could be stress;
- there could be an ergonomically problematic work place;
- there could be a history of injury;
- there could be a malformation of the spine;
- there could be a tumour;
- there could be an inflammation;
- there could be many other specific diseases;
- there could be relationship problems, etc., etc.

Of course, the acupuncturists will claim that, during an acupuncture session, they will pick up on some of these issues. However, in my experience, this is little more than wishful thinking. And even if they did identify other dimensions of the patient's complaint, what can they do about it? They can (and often do) give rather amateur advice. This may be meant kindly but it is rarely optimal and never professional.

And what about conventional practitioners, aren't they even worse? True, often there is much room for improvement. But at least the concept of multifactorial conditions and treatments has been deeply ingrained in everyone who has been through medical school. We learn that symptoms/complaints/conditions/diseases are almost invariably multifactorial; they have many causes and contributing factors which can interact in complex ways. Therefore, responsible physicians always consider treating patients in multifactorial ways. In the case of our neck pain patient, this means that:

- the stress might require treatment, for instance via a relaxation programme;
- the work place might need the input of an occupational therapist;
- in case of an old injury, a referral to a physiotherapist might be required;
- specific conditions might need to be seen by a range of medical specialists;

- muscular tension could be reduced by a massage therapist;
- relationship problems might require the help of a psychologist, etc., etc.

Obviously, not all of this is necessary in each and every case. But at least these possibilities should be considered. In conventional medicine, the concept of a professional multidisciplinary approach is well established, and referrals to other healthcare professionals are a common feature.

By contract, SCAM practitioners claim to be holistic and some might even be aware of the complexity of their patients' symptoms. But, at best, they have an amateur approach to this complexity by issuing more or less well-suited advice. They are not adequately trained to deal with the complexity of most conditions, and they rarely refer their patients to conventional healthcare professionals.

If this is so, why do so many SCAM practitioners claim to be holistic? The answer is simple, in my view: the claim is attractive to consumers and therefore good for business.

3.4. Conspiracy Theories or Paranoia?

Conspiracy theories are notions suggesting that someone is conspiring to create a situation regarded as harmful. In SCAM, conspiracy theories abound [Box 10].

Box 10
Popular conspiracy theories of SCAM supporters

- Big Pharma is determined to maximise their profits at the expense of public health.
- The 'medical establishment' is suppressing information about the benefits of SCAM.
- Vaccinations are known to be harmful but are nevertheless being forced on to our children.
- Drug regulators are in the pocket of the pharmaceutical industry.
- Doctors accept bribes for prescribing dangerous drugs.
- Critics of SCAM are paid by interested parties to denounce it.

A real-life example might explain this better. In a 2016 article entitled 'Bring the Criminals to Justice',[14] a prominent US homeopath protested the rulings by the UK Advertising Standards Authority and the US Federal Trade Commission disallowing the advertising of unsubstantiated claims for homeopathy:[15]

> It's time to hold these people accountable. There are laws in every country against officials taking bribes and malfeasance in office. Write to your legislators and demand that they investigate and bring these criminals to justice. Send them the links to hundreds of homeopathy studies, including disease prevention with homeopathy, at the end of this article. Tell them that the regulatory agencies are protecting Pharma profits, not the public. Meanwhile, let us insist that pharmaceutical drugs be labeled honestly, like this: 'This drug was tested by the same company that profits from it, and which company has been fined millions of dollars in the past for lying about test results. This drug does not cure any medical condition, but only suppresses symptoms which may ultimately make the patient sicker. This drug has already killed or injured X number of people.'

An even more extreme example of a SCAM practitioner plagued by conspiracy theories is the late R.G. Hamer, the founding father of 'Germanic (or German) New Medicine'.[16] Hamer had his medical licence revoked after he was found guilty of malpractice. Subsequently, he continued treating patients as a 'Heilpraktiker' (German non-medically qualified healing practitioner). He has been in court many times, sentenced repeatedly and imprisoned at least twice. Here is what he claims: ...*I do not even believe in the holocaust... I also do*

---

[14] http://hpathy.com/editorials/bring-the-criminals-to-justice/.
[15] https://www.ftc.gov/news-events/press-releases/2016/11/ftc-issues-enforcement-policy-statement-regarding-marketing.
[16] http://www.germannewmedicine.ca/.

not believe that man was on the moon and, much worse, that the Twin Towers were brought down by Arabs, but hardly anybody believes that today...

Hamer's treatments have been associated with several deaths. The most recent case has been reported in an Austrian newspaper:[17]

> An Italian couple apparently had refused to let her daughter's leukaemia be treated with conventional medicine (which usually is life-saving in this condition) but insisted that she receives Hamer's methods of cancer therapy (which are not evidence-based). They therefore took her to a Swiss clinic where she apparently received cortisol and vitamins. After the interventions of Italian doctors, the parents were forbidden to take charge of their daughter's care. Meanwhile, however, the daughter, Eleonora Bottaro from Padova, had reached the age of 18 and was therefore legally allowed to decide about her treatments. She opted to continue the treatment in the Swiss clinic and died of her leukaemia in mid-August.

Hamer also claimed that conventional medicine is guilty of the *'most hideous crime in the whole history of mankind'*. He alleged that Jews have killed around two billion people with morphine, chemotherapy and radiation.

Conspiracy theories seem to be particularly common in the realm of homeopathy. Take this US website,[18] for instance, which states:

> Homeopathic remedies have no side effects. That's a great thing. On the other hand, every drug comes with lots of side effects. And then, you can get in a vicious cycle where you keep taking (or being prescribed) more and more drugs to deal with more and more side effects. In time, this often

---

[17] http://derstandard.at/2000043742380/18-Jaehrige-starbEltern-verweigerten-krebskranker-Tochter-Therapie.

[18] http://devtome.com/doku.php?id=the_natural_superiority_of_homeopathy_and_the_conspiracy_against_you_finding_out.

leads to emergency 'live saving' surgery. When they are successful and the patient doesn't die on the operating table, everyone praises modern medicine for saving those millions of lives, all the while ignoring that the reason those millions of surgeries were needed in the first place, was due to those allegedly wonderful and so-called scientifically proven drugs. Plus, many times, these surgeries aren't truly needed. If the patient would simply quit taking the drugs, the body could, often, heal itself from life threatening conditions...

Homeopathy is much more well known in Europe and various other nations than it is known in the United States. There is a huge medical conspiracy against the use of homeopathy and other medical modalities that threaten the financial dominance of the current medical industry. The conspiracy extends world-wide, but it is strongest in the USA... This conspiracy is being perpetrated on a conscious level, for going on 200 years.

Such examples could, of course, be extreme exceptions. But, sadly, this does not seem to be the case. In a recent US study[19] the investigators presented people with 6 different conspiracy theories. The one that was most commonly believed was the following: THE FOOD AND DRUG ADMINISTRATION IS DELIBERATELY PREVENTING THE PUBLIC FROM GETTING NATURAL CURES FOR CANCER AND OTHER DISEASES BECAUSE OF PRESSURE FROM DRUG COMPANIES. In total, 37% respondents agreed with this statement, 31% had no opinion on the matter, and 32% disagreed. Predictably, the belief in this conspiracy correlated positively with the usage of SCAM.

---

[19] http://jamanetwork.com/journals/jamainternalmedicine/fullarticle/1835348.

Occasionally, one could even get the impression that we are not dealing with conspiracy theories but with overt paranoia. Take this article,[20] for instance:

Given the fact that homeopathy has met with resistance simultaneously on multiple fronts, many are wondering if this is an organized effort. Dr. Larry Malerba, who has practiced homeopathic medicine for more than 25 years, says that he has never witnessed this level of antipathy toward holistic medicine before:

'When one considers the broad array of recent anti-homeopathy activities that cross international borders, it would be naïve to think that there wasn't a common motivating influence. One has to wonder who stands to gain the most from this witch hunt.'

Homeopathy, in particular, is a thorn in the side of Pharma because of the fact that its unique medicines are FDA regulated, safe, inexpensive, and can't be patented. Malerba asked the question,

'Could it be that the media is missing the larger story here, that a powerful medical monopoly is seeking to destroy one of its most successful competitors?'

In India, where homeopathy enjoys tremendous popularity, there are an estimated 250 thousand homeopathic practitioners. Indian homeopath, Dr Sreevals G Menon, seems to agree that there is something fishy going on. He recently wrote:

'The renewed and more vigorous attack on the efficacy of homoeopathy as a curative therapy picked up internationally by the media is nothing but a sinister pogrom by the powerful pharmaceutical corporations the world over.'

...Homeopathic supporters have long suspected that Pharma is secretly funding skeptic organizations. It appears that Pharma astroturfs by taking advantage of skeptic

---

[20] http://www.greenmedinfo.com/blog/pharma-trying-eliminate-homeopathic-competition-1.

organizations that have strong anti-holistic medicine beliefs, encouraging them to spread false information about homeopathy.

But questions remain. Does this constitute an anti-democratic assault on freedom of medical choice? Are media outlets that have been manipulated by corporate medical interests feeding false information to consumers? Why is an increasingly popular medical therapy known for its long track record of safety suddenly receiving so much negative attention?...

It seems that the current popularity of SCAM is to a large extend driven by the conviction that there is a sinister plot by 'the establishment', aimed at preventing people from benefiting from the wonders of SCAM. But where is the evidence for a conspiracy against SCAM? In the many years of researching this area, I have never come across any. On the contrary, the pharmaceutical industry—Big Pharma is the object of a most popular conspiracy theory—seems all too keen to jump on to the alternative bandwagon and maximise their profit by selling SCAM products. Similarly, universities, hospitals, charities and other organisations in health care are currently bending over backwards to accommodate as much SCAM as they possibly can get away with. And they do this despite an embarrassing lack of convincing evidence supporting the treatments in question. To see a conspiracy against SCAM in this trend would therefore be odd.

The closer we look, the more we arrive at the conclusion that the conspiracy against SCAM is a figment of the imagination of those who believe in SCAM. They seem to long for an explanation why their favourite therapy is not more generally accepted than it already is. Cognitive dissonance seems to prevent them from considering that the lack of evidence has anything to do with this situation. Consequently, they prefer to invent a conspiracy theory. If one wanted to be sarcastic, one could even postulate that these notions merely show that SCAM is ineffective in treating paranoia.

3.5. Is SCAM a Cult?

The more I think about this question, the more it makes sense. A cult can be defined not just in a religious context, but also as a non-scientific method claimed by its originator to have exclusive or exceptional power in curing disease. Seen from this perspective, much of SCAM does indeed resemble a cult.

One characteristic of a cult is the unquestioning commitment of its members to the usually bizarre ideas of an iconic leader or guru [Box 11].

Box 11
Cultish adherence of SCAM
proponents to their gurus

- Homeopaths rarely question the doctrines of Hahnemann. On the contrary, to them Hahnemann is the undisputed master.
- Chiropractors seldom doubt even the most ridiculous assumptions of their founding father, D.D. Palmer, who is uncritically worshipped.
- Osteopaths admire Andrew Still, who invented their SCAM and is never questioned.
- Reiki healers blindly follow the received wisdom of their master, Mikao Usui.
- Bach flower therapists admire the bizarre intuitions of Edward Bach who discovered the magic of bottling the healing energy of flowers.
- Bowen therapists worship Thomas Ambrose Bowen, whose 'gift of God' is the basis for their therapeutic approach.
- Alexander teachers unquestionably adopt the teachings of F.M. Alexander, the Australian actor who cured his chronic laryngitis by changing his movement habits.
- Anthroposophical doctors worship Rudolf Steiner, who dreamt up his mystical illusions of anthroposophic medicine.

The cult leader is idealised and not accountable to anyone; he cannot be proven wrong by logical arguments nor by scientific data. He is quite simply immune to any form of scrutiny from inside the cult. Those who dare to disagree with his dogma are expelled, punished or defamed.

Cults persuade their members that nobody outside the cult can be trusted; cults indoctrinate their members into unconditional submission and unquestioning obedience. Likewise, SCAM fanatics believe that anyone criticising SCAM is mistaken and allow themselves to be systematically misinformed to the extent that reality becomes invisible and make-believe becomes reality. They unquestioningly trust in their master, in what they have been told, in what they have read in their cult-books, and in what they have learnt from their cult-peers. The effects of this concerted brainwash can be dramatic: the powers of discrimination vanish, critical questions become impossible, and no amount of evidence can dissuade the SCAM fanatic from abandoning even the most indefensible concepts. Criticism within the group thus becomes unthinkable.

Cults need a mantra, a set of notions that can be repeated endlessly to convince the world of their worth. In SCAM, there is no shortage of possible mantras:

- SCAM is holistic (see section 3.3).
- SCAM is natural (see section 5.1).
- SCAM tackles the root causes (see section 3.1).
- SCAM is the victim of persecution (see section 3.4).
- SCAM has stood the test of time (see section 5.1).

Cults are static; they do not change, make progress or learn from evidence, experience, mistakes, etc. During the last decades, centuries or millennia, homeopathy, chiropractic, acupuncture, energy healing, etc. failed to make any real progress or breakthrough discoveries. Hahnemann, for instance, would pass any exam for homeopathy today. The absurdity of this fact becomes clear if we try to imagine how any of the great physicians of the seventeenth century would fare in any medical exam today.

A popular excuse for the lack of progress in SCAM is that there is no research and no funds to initiate research. This, however, is merely another myth. There are now hundreds of studies of homeopathy or chiropractic, and dozens of energy-healing, for instance. The trouble is not so much the paucity of such research but its findings! The totality of the reliable evidence in each of these areas fails to show that the therapy in question is efficacious. The SCAM cults must supress or defame such evidence because failing to do so would lead to their demise.

Like religious cults, many forms of SCAM promote an elitist concept. Cult-members become convinced of their superiority, based not on rational considerations but on irrational creed. This phenomenon has a range of consequences. For instance, it leads to the isolation of the cult-member from the outside world. Critics of the cult tend to be pitied because they are unable to comprehend the subtleties of the cult's gospel and are thus not taken seriously. For cult-members, external criticism, i.e. criticism from outside the cult, is thus by definition invalid and can be ignored.

Like members of religious cults, SCAM enthusiasts tend to be on a mission. They use any conceivable means to recruit new converts. For instance, they try to convince family, friends and acquaintances of their belief in their particular SCAM at every possible occasion. They also try to operate on a political level for the benefit of their cult. They cherry-pick data, often argue emotionally rather than rationally, and studiously ignore all arguments which contradict their belief system.

In their isolation from society, cult-members tend to assume that outside the cult there is little worthy of their consideration. Similarly, enthusiasts of SCAM often think that their treatment is the only true method of healing. Therapies, concepts and facts which are not cult-approved are systematically defamed, supressed or ignored. An example is the notion of Big Pharma which is employed regularly in SCAM (see previous section). No reasonable person assumes that the pharmaceutical industry smells of roses; however, the exaggerated and systematic denunciation of this industry and its well-documented achievements is a characteristic of virtually all branches of SCAM.

Any spark of doubt or critique in the cult-member is extinguished by the highly effective and incessant flow of mis-information and uncritical promotion. A simple way of demonstrating this phenomenon is, for instance, to analyse the books that are currently being published on SCAM. At present, Amazon UK offers over 50,000 such volumes. I have not read them all, of course, but I estimate that less than 1% is even remotely critical of SCAM—and the authors of this 1% are certainly not members of the SCAM-cult.

3.6. Non-Communication

It has often been commented that SCAM practitioners and conventional healthcare practitioners avoid talking to each other. These are the words of an oncologist with 10 years of experience:[21]

> What do an oncologist and an alternative therapist talk about when a patient like Ainscough dies? Do we defend our individual art, ponder medical ethics or credit individual autonomy above all else? I asked this question of several doctors and the answer was unequivocal. 'We don't talk.' As in, we never talk. Oncologists and alternative health practitioners move in different spheres though plenty of evidence suggests we end up looking after the same patients. When I discover (usually belatedly) that my patient endured the broken promise of an unproven cure, I feel dejected. The more expensive, extreme or exotic the treatment the messier seems the ending.
>
> I have little expectation that someone who would sell false hope to a vulnerable patient would talk me through their reasons why. I once ran into a licensed doctor who oversaw $500 vitamin infusions for cancer patients. The moment when we discovered what the other did was awkward to say the least. My expression asked, 'Why?' I saw him struggle with the answer before he said, 'Because patients want it.' There was no common ground for a conversation and we slid away into the crowd.
>
> Does the natural therapist, coffee enema prescriber or wave therapy expert ever discuss patient care with an oncologist? Not in my experience. There is never written correspondence or a phone call, not even when a patient is desperately ill and it might help to know if some unconventional treatment has led to reversible toxicity. On the

21   https://www.theguardian.com/commentisfree/2015/mar/03/what-do-doctors-say-to-alternative-therapists-when-a-patient-dies-nothing-we-never-talk?CMP=soc_567.

other hand, I occasionally receive requests for tests that the alternative provided can't sign for. The last one was: 'I need a scan to show which natural therapy will best penetrate the tumor.' I politely declined.

...I know it's often said but I honestly don't consider arrogance a good explanation for why oncologists and alternative practitioners don't talk. I would, however, say that dismay and distrust feature heavily. As does the troubling realization that a doctor can face reprimand for inadvertent error but an alternative practitioner can get away with intentional harm.

It is true, the level of non-communication between conventional and SCAM clinicians is stunning. The above quote offers some explanations for this phenomenon. A further reason is that the two camps quite simply have little to say to each other. They live on different planets, talk different languages and have different perspectives. The one who is regularly short-changed in this triangle is doubtlessly the patient.

So, what can be done about this non-communication?

There is no shortage of SCAM sympathisers who advocate building bridges, finding common ground, discussing common patients, etc. However, I am not sure that this approach, over the many years it has been advocated, has been productive or is in the best interest of the patient. Its outcome is usually some type of integration where effective treatments are diluted with dubious ones (see section 5.5). This inevitably renders health-care not more but less effective, and patients, instead of benefiting, are yet again short-changed.

But, what is the solution?

I am not sure that I know the answer. Yet, I am convinced that, to find it, SCAM practitioners need to join the planet of reality, speak the language of reason and share the perspective of evidence-based medicine. I know, it sounds politically incorrect, but I do feel that any truly constructive communication and cooperation between the two camps must take place based on reality rather than wishful thinking.

3.7. Quackademia

When, in 1993, I took up my Exeter post in SCAM research, I also became the head of a centre that conducted courses for SCAM practitioners at the University. After observing what these courses were about, I was so concerned about the centre's lack of academic standards that I swiftly separated my research unit from this activity, discontinued any participation in the centre's teaching, and merely observed the centre's mismanagement leading to its closure about two years later. A full account of this remarkable but sorry tale is provided in my memoir.

In the years that followed, there was a proliferation of SCAM courses in the UK and elsewhere. In 2004, I therefore led an investigation into SCAM courses offered at higher education institutions in the UK. All such institutions listed in a guide as offering SCAM courses were asked to send their written material. Of 25 institutions contacted, 22 responded and 20 information packs could be evaluated according to predefined criteria. Much like the Exeter course mentioned above, these courses seemed not just devoid of science, they even seemed to teach a bizarre form of anti-science. Yet, the students would, at the end of it, receive a 'Bachelor of Science' (BSc) degree. We concluded that many UK higher education institutions are offering SCAM courses of doubtful value and academic calibre.[22]

If one wanted to run a BSc course in, for instance, homeopathy of acceptable academic standard, one would need to teach the students the following essentials about the subject:

- the basics of the scientific method;
- the implausibility of the axioms of homeopathy;
- the largely negative clinical evidence for homeopathy;

---

[22]   Ernst, E., Schmidt, K. Courses in complementary medicine at institutions of higher education in the United Kingdom, Int J Naturopathic Med, 2004; 1: 59–62.

- the reasons why, despite these facts, homeopathy was currently popular.

This means that, at the end of such a BSc course, the student would be well-informed why homeopathy was obsolete nonsense. In reality, however, all these courses were aimed at achieving the opposite.

- They were designed mainly for SCAM practitioners who wanted to get a science degree for boosting their respectability.
- They were taught mainly by SCAM practitioners who were unable to do anything other than promote their trade.
- They were devoid of solid science and full of anti-scientific sentiments.
- They failed to teach critical assessment and promoted uncritical thinking.
- Their academic standard was embarrassingly low.

Not least thanks to the efforts of leading rational thinkers like David Colquhoun, this proliferation of 'quackademia' in the UK stopped. In 2007, he published his influential article entitled 'Science Degrees without Science' in *Nature*:

> ...Things such as golf-course management are honest. They do what it says on the label. That is quite different from awarding BSc degrees in subjects that are not science at all, but are positively anti-science. In my view, they are plain dishonest. One sad consequence of this is the enormous harm it does to the reputations of the 16 post-1992 universities that run CAM degrees in their very proper wish to be recognized as comparable institutions to the older universities. A few older universities also have departments that teach anti-science as fact (for example, complementary medicine groups at the Universities of Southampton and York and the Open University CAM course) but at least they don't award degrees in the subject.
>
> Why don't regulators prevent BSc degrees in anti-science? The Quality Assurance Agency for Higher Educa-

tion (QAA) claims that 'We safeguard and help to improve the academic standards and quality of higher education in the UK.' It costs taxpayers £11.5 million (US$22 million) annually. It is, of course, not unreasonable that governments should ask whether universities are doing a good job. But why has the QAA not noticed that some universities are awarding BSc degrees in subjects that are not, actually, science?...[23]

Meanwhile, in the US, similar problems with 'quackademia' emerged, as this remarkable comment by Donald Marcus points out:

A detailed review of curriculums created by 15 institutions that received educational grants from the National Center for Complementary and Alternative Medicine (NCCAM) showed that they failed to conform to the principles of evidence based medicine. In brief, they cited many poor quality clinical trials that supported the efficacy of alternative therapies and omitted negative clinical trials; they had not been updated for 6–7 years; and they omitted reports of serious adverse events associated with CAM therapies, especially with chiropractic manipulation and with non-vitamin, non-mineral dietary supplements such as herbal remedies. Representation of the curriculums as 'evidence based' was inaccurate and unjustified. Similar defects were present in the curriculums of other integrative medicine programs that did not receive educational grants...

A re-examination of the integrative medicine curriculums reviewed previously showed that they were essentially unchanged since their creation in 2002–03... Why do academic centers that are committed to evidence based medicine and to comparative effectiveness analysis of treatments endorse CAM? One factor may be a concern about jeopardizing income from grants from NCCAM, from

---

[23]   https://www.ncbi.nlm.nih.gov/pubmed/?term=Colquhoun+d%2C+Science+degrees+without+the+science%2C+nature.

CAM clinical practice, and from private foundations that donate large amounts of money to integrative medicine centers. Additional factors may be concern about antagonizing faculty colleagues who advocate and practice CAM, and inadequate oversight of curriculums...

The CAM curriculums violate every tenet of evidence based medicine, and they are a disservice to learners and to the public. It could be argued that, in the name of academic freedom, faculty who believe in the benefits of CAM have a right to present their views. However, as educators and role models they should adhere to the principles of medical professionalism, including 'a duty to uphold scientific standards.' Faculty at health profession schools should urge administrators to appoint independent committees to review integrative medicine curriculums, and to consider whether provision of CAM clinical services is consistent with a commitment to scholarship and to evidence based healthcare.[24]

The notoriously perennial problem of 'quackademia' reveals several things:

- SCAM proponents aim to infiltrate universities.
- This demonstrates their schizophrenic attitude to the 'scientific establishment' in an exemplary fashion: they often are deeply anti-scientific but, at the same time, they like to decorate themselves with a veneer of scientific respectability.
- Many universities are currently run like businesses. They tend to take the money where they can get it. In this climate, issues like scientific credibility tend to become secondary.
- When challenged, universities claim they are supporting free speech, open-mindedness and respectful debate.

---

[24] http://www.bmj.com/content/347/bmj.f5827.

Chapter 4

Research and Researchers

It is a good morning exercise for a research scientist to discard a pet hypothesis every day before breakfast. It keeps him young.
– Konrad Lorenz

4.1. Research Activity in SCAM

For many years, research activity in SCAM has been seemingly buoyant. Since 2013, Medline (the largest electronic data bank for medical papers) listed around 2,000 articles per year in the category of 'complementary alternative medicine'. This must look impressive to lay people. However, compared to other fields of medical research, it is distinctly underwhelming. To view such figures in perspective, we need some comparisons. Let me therefore show you the numbers of Medline-listed articles published in 2016 for a few other areas of conventional medicine:

- Pharmacology: 222,248
- Surgery: 217,494
- Psychology: 83,261
- Internal medicine: 49,747
- Paediatrics: 41,964
- Obstetrics/gynaecology: 23,143
- Rheumatology: 11,449

Now we understand why the 1,933 Medline-listed articles in the category of 'complementary alternative medicine' for 2016 are only seemingly impressive.

But what about specific SCAM therapies? Here are numbers of Medline-listed articles published in 2016 for several specific SCAMs:

- Acupuncture: 1,840
- Herbal medicine: 3,560
- Chiropractic: 459
- Homeopathy: 196
- Aromatherapy: 98
- Naturopathy: 60
- Shiatsu: 111
- Iridology: 0

These figures are not easy to interpret (they also reveal that the umbrella 'complementary alternative medicine' does not catch all SCAM papers). They might indicate, for instance, that certain sections of SCAM are more open to scientific scrutiny than others. Alternatively, they could suggest that some areas are easier to research than others. Or do they demonstrate that, for some areas, there are more research funds and expertise than others? Personally, I suspect all these explanations play a role, but we simply cannot be sure.

If we look a little closer at the research activity in defined SCAM therapies, we are bound to get disappointed. I have recently done this for homeopathy and for acupuncture and reached rather gloomy conclusions:

- Arguably the main research questions of efficacy and safety do not seem to be a priority for SCAM researchers.
- There is an abundance of papers that are data-free and merely thrive on opinion.
- Most of the articles are published in low or very low impact journals.
- Only very few papers are of excellent quality.

You might argue that picking out just two specific SCAMs is not fair; what about SCAM in general? We evaluated all SCAM papers published by US or European authors in 2002.[1] Our analysis showed that, of the 652 articles we found, only 43 were controlled clinical trials, and 51 were surveys. Most articles were of inferior quality.

This plethora of papers reporting surveys is a hallmark of SCAM research, and there is no area of healthcare in which more surveys are being conducted. There is good reason to be critical of this 'survey-mania':[2] most of these articles are of such shoddy quality that they tell us nothing of value. Most of these surveys attempt to evaluate the prevalence of use of SCAM, and it is this type of investigation that I will briefly discuss here.

For such surveys, researchers would design a questionnaire aimed at finding out what percentage of a group of individuals have tried SCAM in the past. Subsequently, the investigators might try to get one or two hundred responses. They then calculate simple descriptive statistics and demonstrate that $xy\%$ (let's assume the figure is 45%) have used SCAM. This finding eventually gets published in one of the many SCAM journals (see section 4.10). Why do I claim that such a result tells us nothing of value? Because the typical SCAM survey has none of the features that would render it a scientific investigation:

1. It lacks an accepted definition of what is being surveyed. There is no generally accepted definition of SCAM, and even if the researchers address specific therapies, they run into problems. Take prayer, for instance—some see this as SCAM, while others would, of course, argue that it is a religious pursuit. Or take herbal medicine—many consumers confuse it with homeopathy, some might think that drinking a cup of tea is herbal medicine (which strictly speaking it is), while others would probably disagree.

---

[1]   https://www.ncbi.nlm.nih.gov/pubmed/?term=giovannini%2C+schmidt%2C+canter%2C+ernst.

[2]   https://www.ncbi.nlm.nih.gov/pubmed/?term=ernst+e+pinch+of+salt.

2. The questionnaires used for such surveys are almost never validated. Essentially, this means that we cannot be sure they quantify what the researchers had intended. We all know that the way we formulate a question can determine the answer. There are uncounted potential sources of bias here, and they are rarely taken into consideration.

3. Enthusiastic researchers of SCAM usually recruit a small convenience sample of participants for their surveys. In other words, they ask a few people who happen to be around to fill their questionnaire. Consequently, there is no way the survey can be representative of the population in question.

4. The typical SCAM survey has a low response rate; sometimes it is not even provided or remains unknown even to the investigators. This means we do not know how most patients/consumers who received but did not fill the questionnaire would have answered. There is good reason to suspect that those who have a certain attitude did respond, while those with a different opinion did not. This self-selection process is likely to produce grossly misleading findings.

So, what? You might ask, what could be the harm in publishing a few flimsy surveys? The answer is that these investigations are regrettably counterproductive because:

- they tend to significantly overestimate the popularity of SCAM,
- they distract money, manpower and attention from the important research questions in this field,
- they give a false impression of a buoyant research activity in SCAM,
- their results are constantly misused.

The last point is crucial, I think. The argument spun around such survey data usually goes roughly as follows:

1. a sizeable percentage of the population uses SCAM,

2. people pay out of their own pockets for these
    treatments,
3. they are satisfied with them — if not, they would not
    pay for them,
4. but why should only those individuals who are rich
    enough to afford it benefit from SCAM? This is not
    fair!
5. Ergo: SCAM SHOULD BE MADE AVAILABLE FOR
    ALL.

In other words, a substantial proportion of research into SCAM
turns out to be pseudo-research (see also next section) which
uses the tools of science not for generating information but for
promoting SCAM.

But SCAM research has a further remarkable feature: the
predominance of positive findings. We have demonstrated that
SCAM journals as well as many individual SCAM researchers
almost never publish negative results.[3] How can this be? The
answer is by adopting a study design which cannot fail to
generate positive results. This allows them to conduct seemingly rigorous trials which can impress consumers and
decision-makers by suggesting that SCAM works wonders
(while, in fact, it doesn't).

Perhaps this is best explained by providing an example. A
recent trial tested the effectiveness of acupuncture as a treatment of cancer-related fatigue.[4] Most cancer patients suffer
from this symptom and it can seriously reduce their quality of
life. Unfortunately, there is little oncologists can do to help, and
therefore SCAM practitioners have a field day claiming that
their interventions are effective. In this trial, cancer patients
who were suffering from fatigue were randomised (meaning
divided according to a random code into two groups) to
receive usual care or usual care plus regular acupuncture. The
researchers then monitored the patients' experience of fatigue

---

[3]   https://www.ncbi.nlm.nih.gov/pubmed?term=ernst%20e%20pittler%20
      nature.
[4]   https://www.ncbi.nlm.nih.gov/pubmed/23109700.

and found that the acupuncture group had less fatigue than the control group. The effect was statistically significant (meaning not due to chance), and an accompanying editorial even called this evidence 'compelling'.[5]

Due to a cleverly over-stated press release, news spread fast, and the study was hailed worldwide as a breakthrough in cancer care. Most commentators felt that research had finally identified an effective therapy for this debilitating symptom which affects so many cancer patients. Hardly anyone seemed to realise that this trial tells us next to nothing about what effects acupuncture has on cancer-related fatigue.

To understand my concern, we need to have a closer look at the trial design. Imagine you have an amount of money A and your friend has the same sum plus another amount B. Who has more money? Simple, it is of course your friend: A+B will always be more than A; and SCAM plus usual care is always better than usual care alone, even if the SCAM is a mere placebo (see section 2.5). Therefore, such 'pragmatic' trials, as they are often called, cannot possibly fail to generate positive results.

Some time ago, we analysed all acupuncture studies with such an "A+B versus B" design.[6] Our hypothesis was that none of these trials would generate a negative result. And—sure enough—it was confirmed by the findings of our analysis.

You might say that, despite these limitations, the above-mentioned acupuncture trial nevertheless provides valuable information. Its authors certainly think so confidently concluding that *acupuncture is an effective intervention for managing the symptom of cancer-related fatigue and improving patients' quality of life.*

The authors of similarly designed SCAM trials would invariably arrive at such positive conclusions. Yet, such studies do not allow conclusions about cause and effect. In other words, they do not show that the therapy in question has

---

[5] https://www.ncbi.nlm.nih.gov/pubmed/23109702.
[6] https://www.ncbi.nlm.nih.gov/pubmed/18626172,

caused the observed result. Acupuncture might be entirely ineffective as a treatment of cancer-related fatigue, and the observed outcome might be due to the extra care and attention, to a placebo response or to other non-specific effects (see section 2.1).

And this is much more than a theoretical concern: rolling out acupuncture across all oncology centres at considerable costs might be entirely the wrong approach for helping these patients. Providing diligent care and compassion could be much more effective as well as less expensive. Adopting acupuncture on a grand scale would also stop us looking for a treatment that is truly effective beyond a placebo—and that surely would not be in the best interests of the patient.

Since we know their result even before the trial has started, such studies are not an honest test of anything. They are not science but thinly disguised pseudo-science with the purpose of being exploited for promotion. They are not just a waste of money and effort, they are dangerous because they produce results that make even useless treatments appear to be effective. In the final analysis, they are therefore unethical.

4.2. Promotion Masquerading as Research

The aim of research, in very simple terms, is to discover the truth. In SCAM, however, it is employed all too often for promotion. This abuse is so very common that many of the SCAM researchers involved in this deceit are not even aware of it. Science, they seem to think, is a tool for marketing products, or for popularising the idea that their particular SCAM is the best thing since sliced bread. To support this statement, I could easily cite hundreds of examples. However, to keep this section manageable, I will focus on just a few recently published papers.

Acupuncture for the US military

This was retrospective analysis[7] of charts from 172 US military personnel who had at least four acupuncture treatments within the last year. The treatment had been administered for a wide range of symptoms, including pain, anxiety and sleep problems. The main outcome measures were prescriptions for opioid medications, muscle relaxants, benzodiazepines and nonsteroidal anti-inflammatory drugs (NSAIDS) in the 60 days prior to the first acupuncture session and in the corresponding 60 days one year later, a symptom-score, ability to perform activities, and quality of life. The results show that all drug prescriptions and symptoms decreased significantly. The authors concluded that *in this military patient population, the number of opioid prescriptions decreased and patients reported improved symptom control, ability to function, and sense of well-being after receiving courses of acupuncture by their primary care physicians.*

This phraseology is intriguing; it implies that the clinical outcomes were the result of the acupuncture treatment without actually stating it. This is perhaps most obvious in the title of the paper: 'Reduction in Pain Medication Prescriptions and Self-Reported Outcomes Associated with Acupuncture in a Military Patient Population'. Yet, there are many explanations for the observed outcomes which are totally unrelated to acupuncture, e.g.:

- the natural history of the conditions that were being treated;
- the conventional therapies which the soldiers received in parallel;
- the regression to the mean;
- social desirability;
- placebo effects.

---

[7]   http://online.liebertpub.com/doi/full/10.1089/acu.2017.1234.

In fact, the results could even be in line with acupuncture causing a delay of clinical improvement; without a control group, we cannot know either way.

SCAM for breast cancer patients

According to its authors, this study[8] was performed *to confirm the benefit of complementary medicine in patients with breast cancer undergoing adjuvant hormone therapy (HT).* A total of 1,561 patients were treated according to international guidelines. They suffered from arthralgia and mucosal dryness due to adjuvant HT. To reduce these symptoms, the patients were treated with a SCAM product containing a combination of several natural ingredients. Outcomes were documented before and four weeks after treatment. Overall, 63% of patients suffering from severe arthralgia and 72% of patients with severe mucosal dryness significantly benefited from the oral combination product. Mean scores of symptoms declined from 4.8 before treatment to 3.2 after four weeks of treatment for arthralgia and from 4.7 before treatment to 3.0 for mucosal dryness. The authors concluded that *this investigation confirms studies suggesting a benefit of complementary treatment with the combination of sodium selenite, proteolytic enzymes and L. culinaris lectin in patients with breast cancer.*

This investigation has too many flaws to mention; here are some of the most obvious ones:

- There was no control group, and therefore we cannot tell whether the patients would not have done just a well (or even better) without taking the SCAM remedy.
- No objective outcome measure was used.
- About 400 patients were not included in the analyses; what happened to them?
- The authors disclose their bias by stating that their aim was *to confirm the benefit of complementary medicine...!*

---

[8]   https://www.ncbi.nlm.nih.gov/pubmed/26709132.

A clinical trial of homeopathy

This study[9] was an *assessment of the clinical effectiveness of homeo-pathic remedies in the alleviation of hay fever symptoms in a typical clinical setting*. The investigator simply observed 8 patients from his private practice using questionnaires at baseline and again after two and four weeks of individualised homeopathic treatment which was given as an adjuvant to conventional treatments. The average symptom scores for the eyes, nose, activity and well-being improved significantly after two and four weeks of homeopathic treatment. The overall average score at baseline was 3.8 and after 14 and 28 days of treatment it had fallen to 1.1 and 1.1 respectively. The author concluded that *individualized homeopathic treatment was associated with significant alleviation of hay fever symptoms, enabling the reduction in use of conventional treatment.*

Here are just four of the many flaws of this study:

- The study design is ill-matched to the research question.
- There is no control group.
- The sample size is tiny.
- The implication that homeopathy had anything to do with the observed outcome is unwarranted.

A systematic review of treatments for shoulder problems

Systematic reviews are aimed at summarising and critically evaluating all the evidence on a specific research question. They are generally considered to be the highest level of evidence and are more reliable than other types of evidence. Therefore, they represent a most useful tool for both clinicians, researchers and consumers (see section 2.1). But there are, of course, exceptions. This systematic review[10] by chiropractors, for instance, was to evaluate the effectiveness of conservative non-drug, non-surgical interventions, either alone or in

---

9   https://www.ncbi.nlm.nih.gov/pubmed/27211328.
10 https://www.ncbi.nlm.nih.gov/pubmed/28554433.

combination, for conditions of the shoulder. The shoulder
conditions addressed were:

- shoulder impingement syndrome (SIS),
- rotator cuff-associated disorders (RCs),
- adhesive capsulitis (AC),
- non-specific shoulder pain.

Twenty-five systematic reviews and 44 RCTs were included in
the analyses. Low- to moderate-quality evidence supported the
use of manual therapies for all four shoulder conditions.
Exercise, particularly combined with physical therapy protocols, was beneficial for SIS and AC. For SIS, moderate evidence
supported several passive modalities. For RC, physical therapy
protocols were found beneficial but not superior to surgery in
the long term. Moderate evidence supported extracorporeal
shockwave therapy for calcific tendinitis RC. Low-level laser
was the only modality for which there was moderate evidence
supporting its use for all four conditions. The authors concluded that *the findings of this literature review may help inform
practitioners who use conservative methods (eg, doctors of chiropractic, physical therapists, and other manual therapists) regarding
the levels of evidence for modalities used for common shoulder
conditions.*

The most striking weakness of this review is its conclusion;
it could have been written even before the project had been
started. It is not based on the data presented and only serves for
promoting chiropractic. Crucially it does not match the stated
aim of this review (*to evaluate the effectiveness of conservative...
interventions*). It appears the authors conducted the review to
promote chiropractic, and when the results turned out not as
they had hoped, they back-peddled to hide this fact as much as
possible.

The question is, how can we protect ourselves from promotion masquerading as research? I only see one solution: we
must sharpen our senses and take SCAM research with more
than a little pinch of salt.

4.3. NCCIAM

The current worldwide boom in SCAM is intimately linked to a centre at the US National Institutes of Health (NIH), the National Center for Complementary and Integrative Health (NCCIAM), formerly called the National Center of Complementary and Alternative Medicine (NCCAM). It was founded in the early 1990s mainly because several pro-SCAM politicians decided that such an institution would be necessary. Initially, the centre had modest funding but, after further lobbying, it received sizeable amounts of cash—around US$ 120 million per year—to pursue a range of activities, including sponsoring research into SCAM. No other institution in the world has ever had more funds for research into SCAM, and the NCCIAM soon became the envy of SCAM researchers globally.

While the level of funding is impressive, the quality of the research sponsored by NCCAIM is sadly the opposite. An example is this recent article;[11] here is a short but telling excerpt from it:

> Researchers led by Richard L. Nahin, PhD, MPH, lead epidemiologist at the NIH's National Center for Complementary and Integrative Health (NCCIH), examined efficacy and safety evidence in 105 randomized controlled trials (RCTs) conducted between January 1966 and March 2016. The review—geared toward primary care physicians as part of the journal's Symposium on Pain Medicine—focused on popular complementary approaches to common pain conditions.
>
> Unlike a typical systematic review that assigns quality values to the studies, the investigators conducted a narrative review, in which they simply looked at the number of positive and negative trials. 'If there were more positives than negatives then we generally felt the approach had some value,' Nahin explained. 'If there were more negatives, we generally felt the approach had less value.' Trials

---

[11] http://jamanetwork.com/journals/jama/article-abstract/2579926.

that were conducted outside of the United States were excluded from the review.

Based on a 'preponderance' of positive vs negative trials, complementary approaches that may offer pain relief include acupuncture and yoga for back pain; acupuncture and tai chi for osteoarthritis of the knee; massage therapy for neck pain; and relaxation techniques for severe head-aches and migraine. Several other techniques had weaker evidence, according to the qualitative assessments, for specific pain conditions (see 'Selected Complementary Health Approaches for Pain'). The treatments were generally safe, with no serious adverse events reported.

The review[12] referred to was published in 2016 and is riddled with many major flaws:

- the safety of SCAM was evaluated based on data from RCTs; yet, it has been shown repeatedly that trials of SCAM often fail to report adverse effects;[13] in any case, much larger samples would have been needed for adequate safety assessments,
- the authors only included RCTs from the US, which must result in a skewed and incomplete picture;
- the discussion of the paper totally lacks any evidence of critical thinking;
- there is no assessment of the quality of the trials included in this review.

The last point is by far the most important. A summary of this nature that fails to consider the often-serious limitations of the primary studies is as good as worthless.

But this is, of course, just one single article from the NCCAIM. It could therefore be a glitch — but sadly, it is not. Some years ago, we evaluated the quality of all the NCCAIM-

---

[12]   http://www.mayoclinicproceedings.org/article/S0025-6196(16)30317-2/fulltext.

[13]   https://www.ncbi.nlm.nih.gov/pubmed/22522273.

sponsored research of four specific SCAMs. Here are the conclusions of our assessments:

Acupuncture

Seven RCTs had a low risk of bias. Numerous methodological shortcomings were identified. Many NCCAIM-funded RCTs of acupuncture have important limitations. These findings might improve future studies of acupuncture and could be considered in the ongoing debate regarding NCCAIM-funding.[14]

Herbal Medicine

This independent assessment revealed a plethora of serious concerns related to NCCAIM studies of herbal medicine.[15]

Energy Medicine

The NCCAIM-funded RCTs of energy medicine are prime examples of misguided investments into research. In our opinion, NCCAIM should not be funding poor-quality studies of implausible practices. The impact of any future studies of energy medicine would be negligible or even detrimental.[16]

Chiropractic

Our review demonstrates that several RCTs of chiropractic have been funded by the NCCAM. It raises numerous concerns in relation to these studies; in particular, it suggests that many of these studies are seriously flawed.[17]

---

[14] *Focus on Alternative and Complementary Therapies*, Volume 17 (1), March 2012: 15–21.
[15] *Perfusion*, 2011, 24: 89–102.
[16] *Focus on Alternative and Complementary Therapies*, Volume 16 (2), June 2011: 106–109.
[17] https://www.ncbi.nlm.nih.gov/pubmed/21207089.

The overall conclusion that seems to emerge from these assessments is that NCCIAM is impressive through the level of funding it receives from US tax-payers. However, the hope of many experts that the centre would stand for good science and rigorous assessments of SCAM was bitterly disappointed. The quality of the NCCIAM-sponsored research is often poor. I therefore agree with another critic who stated: *this politicized branch of the NIH is more concerned with placating the quackophiles than it is with finding useful practices and products that would benefit the public.*[18]

4.4. The Making of a Pseudo-Researcher

Pseudo-scientists in SCAM are foremost recognisable by the fact that they study their subject not with the aim of testing a hypothesis — as scientists are supposed to do — but with the urge to prove the correctness of their prior beliefs and assumptions. The way I see it, there are two pathways towards the career of a pseudo-scientist in SCAM: the epiphany and the gravy train.

Epiphany

The starting point of the epiphany is an impressive personal experience which is often akin to a moment of sudden and great revelation or realisation. I have met hundreds of advocates of homeopathy, and those who talk about their very own epiphany invariably offer impressive stories about how they metamorphosed from being a 'sceptic' — yes, they almost all claim to have been a sceptic — into someone who was completely bowled over by homeopathy. This 'Saulus–Paulus conversion' usually relates to that person's own (or a close friend's) illness which was allegedly cured by homeopathy.

Rachel Roberts, chief executive of the UK Homeopathy Research Institute, provides an excellent example:[19]

---

[18]   http://www.skepdic.com/NCCAM.html.
[19]   https://www.theguardian.com/commentisfree/2010/jul/15/homeopathy-works-scientific-evidence.

I was a dedicated scientist about to begin a PhD in neuro-science when, out of the blue, homeopathy bit me on the proverbial bottom. Science had been my passion since I began studying biology with Mr Hopkinson at the age of 11, and by the age of 21, when I attended the dinner party that altered the course of my life, I had still barely heard of it. The idea that I would one day become a homeopath would have seemed ludicrous. That turning point is etched in my mind. A woman I'd known my entire life told me that a homeopath had successfully treated her when many months of conventional treatment had failed. As a sceptic, I scoffed, but was nonetheless a little intrigued. She confessed that despite thinking homeopathy was a load of rubbish, she'd finally agreed to an appointment, to stop her daughter nagging. But she was genuinely shocked to find that, after one little pill, within days she felt significantly better. A second tablet, she said, 'saw it off completely'. I admit I ruined that dinner party. I interrogated her about every detail of her diagnosis, previous treatment, time scales, the lot. I thought it through logically—she was intelligent, she wasn't lying, she had no previous inclination towards alternative medicine, and her reluctance would have diminished any placebo effect. Scientists are supposed to make unprejudiced observations, then draw conclusions. As I thought about this, I was left with the highly uncom-fortable conclusion that homeopathy appeared to have worked. I had to find out more. So, I started reading about homeopathy, and what I discovered shifted my world for ever. I became convinced enough to hand my coveted PhD studentship over to my best friend and sign on for a three-year, full-time homeopathy training course. Now, as an experienced homeopath, it is 'science' that is biting me on the bottom. I know homeopathy works...

Another poignant example is Susan Samueli. She was reported to have caught a cold while visiting France. Instead of the usual medicines, a friend suggested a homeopathic remedy. She was cured, and became a lifelong advocate of homeopathy and other SCAMs. Her husband, Henry — the billionaire co-founder of Broadcom, the Irvine semiconductor maker — says he was initially sceptical but found the integrative health approach helped him easily shake off colds and flus and kept their children healthy without antibiotics. The Samuelis have recently donated US$ 200 million for SCAM research.[20]

I have heard many strikingly similar accounts. Some of these tales seem a little too tall to be true and might be a trifle exaggerated, but the consistency of the picture that emerges from these stories is nevertheless extraordinary: people get started on a single anecdote which then escalates into an epiphany. Subsequently, they are on a mission of confirming their new-found belief repeatedly. Eventually, they become undoubting and devoted disciples for life.

In no other area of healthcare other than SCAM does the initial anecdote regularly play such a prominent role. People do not become believers in aspirin, beta-blockers or bone marrow transplants based on a 'moment of great revelation'; they start using a therapy because of the evidence. And, if there is a discrepancy between the negative external evidence and their own positive experience (as there clearly is with homeopathy[21, 22]) most people would begin to reflect: what other explanations exist to rationalise the anecdote? Invariably, there are many (placebo, natural history of the condition, concomitant events etc. — see section 2.1).

Gravy train

The second pathway towards becoming a pseudo-scientist is much more profane and could be called the 'gravy train'. Let me try to explain it in the form of a 'story' of a young doctor who jumps on this train to become an ardent homeopath:

---

[20]   http://www.latimes.com/local/lanow/la-me-uc-irvine-donation-20170918-story.html.
[21]   https://www.nhmrc.gov.au/guidelines-publications/cam02.
[22]   http://www.easac.eu/fileadmin/PDF_s/reports_statements/EASAC_Homepathy_statement_web_final.pdf.

After our young doctor — I'll call him Walter, shall I? — had finished medical school, he wanted nothing more than to help and assist needy patients. A chain of coincidences made him take a post in a homeopathic hospital where he worked as a junior clinician alongside several experienced homeopaths. What he saw impressed him: contrary to what he had learnt at medical school, homeopathy seemed to work quite well: patients with all sorts of symptoms told Walter they had benefited from homeopathy.

As his ability to think clearly grew, Walter nevertheless began to wonder: were his patients' improvements really and truly due to the homeopathic remedies, or were these outcomes perhaps caused by the kind and compassionate care he and the other staff provided for their patients? To cut a long story short, when Walter left the hospital to establish his own practice, he knew how to prescribe homeopathics, but he had not become a fully convinced homeopath. Over the following months, Walter made less and less use of homeopathy in his routine practice. Quite frankly, he did not see much success in his homeopathic prescriptions — not until one day, a young woman consulted him; she and her husband had been unsuccessfully trying to have a baby for two years. Now she was getting very frustrated, even depressed, with her childlessness. All tests on her and her husband had failed to reveal any abnormalities. A friend had told her that homeopathy might help, and she had therefore made this appointment to consult a homeopath.

Walter was not convinced that he could help his patient but, in the end, the desperate young woman persuaded him to give it a try. He conducted a full homeopathic history to find the optimal remedy for his patient, gave her an individualised prescription and explained that the effect might take a while. The patient was delighted, felt well cared for by Walter, and seemed full of optimism. Months passed and she returned for several further consultations. But sadly, she failed to get pregnant. About a year later, when all involved had all but given up hope, the test confirmed: she was expecting! Everyone was surprised, not least Walter. This outcome, he reasoned, could not possibly be due to placebo, or the good therapeutic relationship he had been able to establish with his patient. Perhaps it was just a coincidence?

In the town where they lived, news spread quickly that Walter was able to treat infertility with homeopathy. Other women with the same problem liked the idea of having an effective yet risk-free therapy for their infertility problem. Walter thus treated several further infertile women during the next months. Amazingly most of them got pregnant within a year or so. Walter was baffled, such a series of pregnancies could not be a coincidence!

Naturally, the cases that were talked about were the women who had become pregnant. And naturally, these were the patients Walter liked to remember (nobody likes dwelling on their failures). Slowly he became convinced that he was indeed able to treat infertility with homeopathy. He even published a paper in a national homeopathic journal about his successes. In a way, he had hoped that perhaps someone would challenge him and explain where his reasoning that homeopathy had caused the fertility had gone wrong. But the article was greeted with much applause, and he was even invited to speak at several conferences. In short, within a few years, Walter made himself a name for his ability to treat infertility.

Patients now travelled from across the country to see him; some even came from abroad. Walter had become a minor celebrity. Some journalists had even written articles about his amazing skills. He also, one must admit, had started to make very good money; most of his patients were private patients. Life was good. Naturally, all his former doubts about the effectiveness of homeopathic remedies gradually dissolved into thin air. Whenever now someone challenged his findings with arguments like 'Homeopathy is implausible; homeopathics are just placebos; homeopathy is quackery', Walter surprised himself by getting quite angry. How do they dare doubt my data, he thought? The babies are there; nobody can deny their existence — homeopathy is effective!

But there are, of course, much more plausible explanations for Walter's apparent success rate: otherwise healthy women, who don't get pregnant within months of trying, do usually succeed eventually, even without any treatment whatsoever. Walter had struck lucky when this happened a few times after the first patient had consulted him. Had he prescribed non-homeopathic placebos, his success rate would have been the same.

Yes, the two pathways to becoming a pseudo-researcher do have a moral: for clinicians, it is tempting not to adequately rationalise success. If the 'success' then happens repeatedly, clinicians are in danger of becoming deluded, and they almost automatically 'forget' their failures. Over time, this 'confirmation bias', as experts call the phenomenon, will create an increasingly misleading impression and often even a deeply felt conviction.

I am sure that this sort of thing happens often, and it happens not just to SCAM practitioners. It happens to all types of practitioners. This is how ineffective treatments survive for often very long periods. This is how blood-letting survived for centuries. This is how millions of patients get harmed following the advice of their trusted physicians to employ a useless or even dangerous therapy.

To prevent the creation of pseudo-researchers, scientists and clinicians (and everyone else, for that matter) need to systematically learn how to think critically. But even today, courses in critical thinking are rarely part of the university curriculum, certainly not at medical school. I find this most lamentable; in my view, they would be as important as anatomy, physiology or any of the other core subjects in medicine.

4.5. How Can We Differentiate Good from Bad Research?

This is a straightforward, reasonable and often-asked question. It should therefore be easy to answer. As it turns out, however, the distinction is far from easy. In this section, I will provide a few indicators as to what might signify a good and a poor clinical trial of SCAM (other types of research would need somewhat different criteria). So, here is my list of 18 indicators:

1. Author from a respected institution.
2. Article published in a respected journal.
3. A precise research question.
4. Full description of the methods used so that an independent researcher can repeat the study.
5. Randomisation of study participants into experimental and control groups.
6. Use of a placebo in the control group where in line with the research question.
7. Blinding of patients.
8. Blinding of investigators, including clinicians administering the treatments and scientists evaluating the findings.
9. Clear definition of a primary outcome measure.
10. Sufficiently large sample size.
11. Adequate statistical analyses.
12. Presentation of the data such that an independent assessor can check them.
13. Understandable write-up of the entire study.
14. A discussion that shows critical thinking and puts the study into the context of all the important previous work in this area.
15. Self-critical analysis of the study design, conduct and interpretation of the results.
16. Cautious conclusions which are strictly based on the data presented.
17. Full disclosure of ethics approval, informed consent, funding sources and conflicts of interest.
18. Up-to-date list of references that also includes papers that contradict the authors' findings.

Yes, this list is technical and, I must admit, quite boring. What might be more fun is to name some features of a clinical trial that signify a poor quality study. This could be a helpful guide for reading such publications. So, let's try that; here is my list of 17 indicators suggesting a poor clinical trial:

1. Article published in one of the many dodgy SCAM journals (or in a book, blog or similar, see section 4.10).
2. Single author.
3. Author(s) known to be proponents of the treatment tested.
4. Authors who have previously published nothing but positive studies of the therapy in question.
5. Lack of plausible rationale for the study or the therapy.
6. Stated aim of the study is 'to demonstrate the effectiveness of...' (clinical trials are for **testing**, not demonstrating effectiveness or efficacy).
7. Stated aim 'to establish the effectiveness **and safety** of...' (even large trials are usually far too small to establish the safety of an intervention; other types of research are needed for investigating safety).
8. Text is full of mistakes, e.g. spelling, grammar, etc.
9. Sample size is tiny.
10. Pilot study reporting anything other than the feasibility of a definitive trial.
11. Methods not described in sufficient detail for an independent replication of the study.
12. Mismatch between aim, method and conclusions of the study.
13. Results presented only as a graph rather than figures which others can recalculate.
14. Statistical approach inadequate or not sufficiently detailed.
15. Discussion without critical input.
16. Lack of disclosures of ethics approval, funding-source or conflicts of interest.
17. Conclusions which are not based on the results.

The problem here (as with my first list above) is that one would need to write an entire book to render it more comprehensible. Without further detailed explanations, the issues raised could remain rather abstract or nebulous, particularly for people who rarely read scientific papers. Therefore, let me provide just three examples that make some of these points a little clearer.

My first example[23] is a trial that, according to its authors, tested the efficacy and safety of combining shiatsu with the drug amitriptyline to treat headaches in a single-blind study. Subjects with a diagnosis of primary headache were randomised to receive one of the following treatments:

- shiatsu plus amitriptyline;
- shiatsu alone;
- amitriptyline alone.

The treatments lasted three months. The primary end point was the proportion of patients experiencing at least a 50% reduction in headache days. A total of 11 patients were allocated to the shiatsu plus amitriptyline group, 13 to shiatsu alone, and 13 to amitriptyline alone. The results show that all the three groups improved and there was no between-group difference in the primary end point. Shiatsu (alone or in combination) was superior to amitriptyline in reducing the number of pain killers taken per month. Seven subjects reported adverse events, all attributable to amitriptyline, while no side effects were related to shiatsu. The authors concluded that *shiatsu is a safe and potentially useful alternative approach for refractory headache. However, there is no evidence of an additive or synergistic effect of combining shiatsu and amitriptyline.*

Applying my above checklist, we find that:

- the study lacked a proper rationale,
- there was no adequate placebo control,
- the aim of testing the safety of the intervention is not realistic,
- the sample size was tiny,
- the trial was labelled to be pilot study,
- the conclusion is not based on the results of the study.

---

[23]   https://www.ncbi.nlm.nih.gov/pubmed/28283760.

My second example[24] is a study that compared the efficacy of Emotional Freedom Technique (EFT, a SCAM that involves acupoint stimulation) with that of Cognitive-Behavioural Therapy (CBT) in reducing adolescent anxiety. Sixty-three students with moderate to high anxiety were randomly assigned to one of three groups:

- CBT ($n = 21$),
- EFT ($n = 21$),
- or waitlist control ($n = 21$).

Students assigned to the CBT or EFT treatment groups received three individual sessions. EFT participants showed significant reduction in anxiety levels compared with the waitlist control group; CBT participants did not differ significantly from the EFT or control. The authors concluded that *EFT is an efficacious intervention to significantly reduce anxiety for high-ability adolescents.*

Based on my checklist, we find that this investigation:

- was published in a SCAM journal,
- had no proper rationale,
- did not use an adequate placebo control,
- had a small sample size,
- was a pilot study,
- had conclusions that were not based on the results.

My third example is a study[25] that was conducted *to determine if a homeopathic syrup was effective in treating cold symptoms in preschool children.* Children suffering from a cold were randomised to receive a commercial homeopathic cold syrup or placebo. Parents administered the study medication as needed for three days. The primary outcome was change in symptoms one hour after each dose. Data on 957 doses of study medication in 154 children were analysed. There was no significant

---

[24]   http://online.liebertpub.com/doi/abs/10.1089/acm.2015.0316?journalCod e=acm.
[25]   https://www.ncbi.nlm.nih.gov/pubmed/27912951.

difference in improvement in the primary outcome measure. However, an analysis of secondary end points found some benefit of the homeopathic preparation over placebo. The authors concluded that *the homeopathic syrup appeared to be effective in reducing the severity of cold symptoms in the first day after beginning treatment.*

There are so many problems with this study that I find it difficult to choose the most crucial ones. According to my checklist, the most significant one is number 17: the study had a clearly defined primary end point which was not affected by the homeopathic treatment which undeniably makes the study a negative trial. A correct conclusion therefore would be that **the homeopathic syrup failed to affect the primary outcome measure of this study. Therefore, the trial did not produce any evidence to assume that the experimental treatment was efficacious.**

Even though these discussions are unavoidably technical, I hope that those who are novices to reading clinical trials of SCAM might be able to use my checklist to tell rigorous clinical trials from flimsy studies. My final advice is neither technical nor complicated: if it sounds too good to be true, it probably is.

4.6. Scientific Misconduct

Any action that wilfully compromises the integrity of scientific research could be scientific misconduct. This can range from misinterpretation of data to overt cheating. Perhaps the most obvious form of scientific misconduct is intentional fabrication of scientific data.

It is indisputable that scientific misconduct causes severe damage to science and the public. In healthcare, it also has the potential to harm patients as well as society at large. If, for instance, a certain treatment is accepted into routine care based on fabricated data, this could put patients' lives at risk. If that treatment is being paid for by the system, society will be deprived of funds that are badly needed elsewhere.

Sadly, scientific misconduct exists in all types of research. In SCAM, I have seen more of it than I care to remember. To write about it is, however, tricky. Libel laws are such that detailing concrete cases might turn out to be a costly affair, even if one is victorious. In this chapter, I will therefore focus on two examples of historic, well-documented cases.

Sigmund Rascher (1909–1945)

I first became aware of Dr Sigmund Rascher's work when, in the early 1980s, I was studying the influence of body temperature on the flow properties of blood at the University of Munich. I then learnt of Rascher's unspeakably cruel and grossly unethical experiments in the Dachau concentration camp exposing prisoners to extreme hypothermia. Many of Rascher's 'volunteers' had lost their lives.[26, 27]

I had hoped to never again hear of this monster of a physician—yet, many years later, I once more came across Rascher in the context of my research into SCAM. Rascher had been brought up in Rudolf Steiner's anthroposophical tradition, and his very first 'research' project was on an alternative blood test advanced by a friend of Rascher who had developed a bizarre diagnostic method using copper-chloride crystallisation of blood and other materials. This copper-chloride bio-crystallisation (CCBC) became the subject of Rascher's doctoral dissertation in Munich.

The CCBC involves a visual evaluation of copper crystals which form in the presence of blood or other fluids, a method which is wide open to interpretation and bias. The CCBC is still used by some anthroposophical or homeopathic doctors today. This current article,[28] for instance, explains: *A few drops of blood are brought to crystallisation with copper chloride in a climate chamber. Decades of experience allow a very early diagnosis of all functional weaknesses of the organs and glands as well as of cancer.*

---

[26] https://www.ncbi.nlm.nih.gov/pubmed/2184357.
[27] https://www.amazon.co.uk/Fall-House-Rascher-bizarre-SS-doctor-ebook/dp/B00MBOFX5K/ref=sr_1_1?s=books&ie=UTF8&qid=1450633403&sr=1-1&keywords=sigmund+rascher.
[28] http://www.dr-nawrocki.de/diagnoseKristAmsat.html.

Cancer can often be detected earlier than with any other method. (My own translation from German.)

The reference to 'decades of experience' is more than a little ironic, because the evidence suggesting that the CCBC might generate valid findings rests exclusively on Rascher's work from the 1930s; to the best of my knowledge no other 'validation' of the CCBC has ever become available. With his initial thesis, Rascher had produced amazingly positive results and he subsequently lobbied to get an official research grant for testing the CCBC's usefulness, specifically for diagnosing cancer.

Most of Rascher's later research — some of it on SCAM — was conducted in the Dachau concentration camp with the active support of Heinrich Himmler. In 1941, a research unit was established in 'Block 5' of the camp which, according to Rascher's biographer, included Rascher's department together with a homeopathic research unit.

Today, experts agree that Rascher's research, including his early work on the CCBC, was fraudulent, and his data were totally or partly fabricated. It seems that his MD thesis on the CCBC set him off on a lifelong career of research misconduct.

Shortly before the end of the Third Reich, Rascher lost the support of Himmler and was imprisoned for a string of offences which were largely unrelated to his 'research'. As a prisoner, he was eventually brought back to the place of his worst atrocities, the concentration camp of Dachau. Days before the liberation of the camp by the US forces, Rascher was executed; it is believed that this happened on direct orders of Himmler who wanted to silence an important witness of the medical experiments conducted under his guidance and protection.

David Horrobin (1939–2003)

In SCAM, the line between wishful thinking and overt fraud seems often blurred, as my second example demonstrates. One of the best-selling supplements is evening primrose oil (EPO). It is being promoted for a wide range of conditions, including eczema. Yet, our Cochrane review[29] *concluded that oral borage oil and evening primrose oil lack effect on eczema; improvement was similar to respective placebos used in trials. Oral BO and EPO are not effective treatments for eczema.*

The notion that EPO is effective for eczema and several other conditions was originally promoted by the researcher turned entrepreneur, D.F. Horrobin. In the 1980s, Horrobin began to sell EPO supplements without having conclusively demonstrated their safety and efficacy. This action led to confiscations and felony indictments in the US. As chief executive of Scotia Pharmaceuticals, Horrobin obtained licences for several EPO-preparations which were later withdrawn for lack of efficacy. Charges of mismanagement and fraud led to Horrobin being ousted as CEO by the board of the company. Later, Horrobin published a positive meta-analysis of EPO for eczema where he included findings of seven of his own unpublished and therefore not peer-reviewed studies with apparently positive results, but excluded the negative results of the largest published trial.

The evidence for EPO is not just negative for eczema. To the best of my knowledge, there is not a single disease or symptom for which it demonstrably works. Our own review[30] of the data concluded that EPO *has not been established as an effective treatment for any condition.*

Horrobin clearly misled patients, healthcare professionals, scientists, regulators, decision makers and businessmen. This caused unnecessary expense and it obstructed research efforts and progress in a multitude of areas.

---

[29]   https://www.ncbi.nlm.nih.gov/pubmed/23633319.
[30]   https://www.amazon.co.uk/Desktop-Guide-Complementary-Alternative-Medicine/dp/0723433836.

Society for Integrative Oncology

I will finish this section by asking my readers a question: does the following current case amount to scientific misconduct, or is it merely an unintended error?

The 'Clinical Practice Guidelines on the Use of Integrative Therapies as Supportive Care in Patients Treated for Breast Cancer' published by the 'Society for Integrative Oncology (SIO) Guidelines Working Group'[31] aim to *inform clinicians and patients about the evidence supporting or discouraging the use of specific complementary and integrative therapies for defined outcomes during and beyond breast cancer treatment, including symptom management.* The conclusions of the guidelines stated: *Specific integrative therapies can be recommended as evidence-based supportive care options during breast cancer treatment.*

The research that led to this conclusion seems rigorous, at least at first sight. A team of researchers defined the treatments they wanted to look at, searched for randomised controlled trials (RCTs), evaluated their quality, extracted their results and combined them into an overall verdict. Based on the findings of their review, they then issued specific recommendations which, I thought, were baffling in several respects (see my comments in square brackets). Here I will focus on just three of the SIO's recommendations dealing with acupuncture:

1. *Acupuncture can be considered for treating anxiety concurrent with ongoing fatigue...* [only one RCT cited in support.]
2. *Acupuncture can be considered for improving depressive symptoms in women suffering from hot flashes...* [only two RCTs cited in support.]

31

https://www.ncbi.nlm.nih.gov/pmc/articles/PMC4411539/#CIT0057

3. *Acupuncture can be considered for treating anxiety con-current with ongoing fatigue... [only one RCT cited in support.]*

One or two studies as a basis for far-reaching guidelines must be a concern, particularly as the RCTs in question are not nearly of the calibre to allow firm conclusions. Many other recommendations made in the document seem to be based on similarly 'liberal' interpretations of the evidence. More doubts emerge when reading the following collective statement about the authors' conflicts of interest: *There are no financial conflicts of interest to disclose. We note that some authors have conducted/authored some of the studies included in the review.* This seems surprising: most of the guidelines' authors earn their living by practising integrative medicine.

Honest errors or scientific misconduct? You decide!

4.7. Nonsensical Research

We have previously discussed why clinical trials should be designed in certain ways to generate reliable results (section 2.1). But adopting a rigorous trial design is by no means a guarantee for producing meaningful research. Even the most rigorously designed study can be utterly nonsensical. Imagine, for instance, a rigorous clinical trial of bungee-jumping for curing ingrown toenails. Does that sound ridiculous? In SCAM, this sort of thing is sadly not a rare event.

Take this randomised, triple-blind, placebo-controlled cross-over trial of homeopathy, for example.[32] Its authors recruited 86 volunteers suffering from 'mental fatigue' and treated them with the homeopathic remedy Kali-Phos 6X or placebo for one week. The results failed to show that the homeopathic medication had any effect.

As we all know, clinical trials are for testing hypotheses. But what is the hypothesis tested here? According to the authors,

---

[32] https://www.ncbi.nlm.nih.gov/pubmed?term=macpherson%20homeopathy.

the aim was to *assess the effectiveness of Kali-Phos 6X for attention problems associated with mental fatigue.* In other words, their hypothesis was that this remedy is effective for treating the symptom of mental fatigue. But this notion is not a scientific hypothesis, it is a foolish conjecture! By way of justification for the RCT in question, the authors inform us that <u>one</u> previous trial had suggested an effect. This might sound alright, but on closer scrutiny it turns out that the study in question did not employ just Kali-Phos but a combined preparation which included Kali-Phos as <u>one of several</u> components. Thus, the authors' 'hypothesis' does not even amount to a hunch. In other words, the entire project failed to make sense. And if we test nonsense, the result can only be nonsense.

My second example is also a trial of a homeopathic product; this time as a treatment for chronic low back pain.[33] The only justification for conducting this RCT was that, according to the authors, the manufacturer of the remedy allegedly knew of a few unpublished case-reports which suggested their remedy was effective. Already a case-report is not convincing; an unpublished one is even less, and an unpublished case-report only known to the manufacturer is next to nothing. A total of 150 patients were randomly allocated to receive either injections with the homeopathic remedy, placebo injections, or no treatment at all. The results show no difference in outcome between the remedy and the placebo group. Anyone with a background in science or even with a minimum of common sense might have predicted that outcome—which is why such nonsensical trials are deplorably wasteful and arguably unethical. Research funds are increasingly scarce, and they must not be spent on nonsensical projects! The money and time should be invested more fruitfully elsewhere. Participants of clinical trials give their cooperation willingly; but if they learn that their efforts have been wasted unnecessarily, they might think twice next time they are asked. Thus, nonsensical

---

[33] https://www.ncbi.nlm.nih.gov/pubmed/22087222.

research projects may have knock-on effects with far-reaching consequences.

My third example is a study of Bach Flower Remedies. Like homeopathic medicines, these remedies are highly diluted and therefore devoid of active molecules. Consequently, the evidence for these treatments is squarely negative: my systematic review[34] analysed the data of all seven RCTs available in 2010. All the placebo-controlled trials failed to demonstrate efficacy, and I concluded that *the most reliable clinical trials do not show any differences between flower remedies and placebos.*

Yet the authors of this study[35] boldly stated that their aim was *to evaluate the effect of Bach Flower Rescue Remedy on the control of risk factors for cardiovascular disease in rats.* A randomised longitudinal experimental study was conducted on 18 rats which were randomly divided into three groups of 6 animals each and dosed with either 200µl of water (group A, control), or 100µl of water with 100µl of Bach Flower Remedy (group B), or 200µl of Bach Flower Remedy (group C) every 2 days, for 20 days. The investigators then measured a wide range of outcomes. No significant differences were found in food intake, faeces weight, urine volume and uric acid levels between groups. Group C had a significantly lower body weight gain than group A and lower glycaemia compared with groups A and B. Groups B and C had significantly higher HDL-cholesterol and lower triglycerides than controls. From this, the authors concluded that *Bach Flower Rescue Remedy was effective in controlling glycaemia, triglycerides, and HDL-cholesterol and may serve as a strategy for reducing risk factors for cardiovascular disease in rats. This study provides some preliminary 'proof of concept' data that Bach Rescue Remedy may exert some biological effects.*

If ever I saw a nonsensical study, it must be this one: nobody has ever claimed that Rescue Remedy modified cardiovascular risk factors. The hypothesis of this trial makes no sense

---

[34] https://www.ncbi.nlm.nih.gov/pubmed/20734279.
[35] https://www.ncbi.nlm.nih.gov/pubmed/25146077.

whatsoever. To test it in rats borders on the ridiculous, in my view.

Clinical trials are tools for testing hypotheses. Like any other tool, they can be abused. One sure way of misusing clinical trials is to employ them for testing implausible hunches or wishful thinking. The result inevitably is nonsense. In SCAM, such nonsense is highly prevalent and causes untold damage:

- It is wastes scarce research funds.
- It betrays the trust of patients.
- It violates research ethics.
- It defames clinical research.

4.8. Too Good to Be True

After reading virtually thousands of SCAM articles, I am often left with an uncomfortably strong feeling that something is badly amiss. The impression I frequently get is that the results are too good to be true. This is perhaps best explained by providing a few examples.

My first example is a placebo-controlled clinical trial[36] aimed at evaluating the effectiveness of a cream based on Bach Flower Remedies (BFR) for alleviating the symptoms of carpal tunnel syndrome (a painful condition where the tendons around the wrist become so tight that they irritate the nerves). Forty-three patients were randomised into three groups:

- placebo ($n = 14$),
- blinded BFR cream ($n = 16$),
- non-blinded BFR cream ($n = 13$).

After 21 days of treatment, significant improvements were observed on self-reported symptom severity favourable to the two BFR groups. The authors of this study concluded that *the proposed BFR cream could be an effective intervention in the management of mild and moderate carpal tunnel syndrome, reducing the severity of symptoms and providing pain relief.*

---

[36]   https://www.ncbi.nlm.nih.gov/pubmed/26456628.

To me, these findings sound far too good to be true. The notion that BFR — normally taken by mouth — which contain no active ingredients, are more than placebos is not plausible. The assumption that BFR work as a cream is even less plausible. Before publication of this paper, the editor of the journal should have asked for the original data and had them re-analysed by an independent statistician. As we cannot do that, our only option is to apply common sense and a healthy dose of scepticism.

My second example relates to wet cupping, a therapy involving superficial injuries to the skin with subsequent application of a vacuum cup over the injured site. This procedure would draw a small amount of blood into the cup, and this visible effect is taken as a sign that the humours or life forces are being restored. The aim of this clinical trial[37] was to evaluate the effectiveness and safety of wet cupping therapy as the sole treatment for persistent non-specific low back pain (PNSLBP). The investigators randomised 80 patients to the cupping group or to a control group. The former group had six wet cupping sessions within two weeks, while the control group had no such treatments. At the end of the intervention and two weeks thereafter, statistically significant differences were noted for pain favouring the cupping group. The authors concluded that *wet cupping is potentially effective in reducing pain and improving disability associated with PNSLBP at least for 2 weeks after the end of the wet cupping period.*

Apart from the numerous weaknesses of the study design, these results seem highly implausible to me. Low back pain has a natural history that is well-studied. We therefore know that most patients do get better regardless of whether we treat them or not. In this study, the control group did not improve at all. This is most unlikely, and one might suspect that this lack of improvement generated the false impression that wet cupping was effective.

---

37   http://online.liebertpub.com/doi/full/10.1089/acm.2015.0065.

The third example concerns an entire area of therapeutics, namely studies of acupuncture made in China, where 100% of all findings are positive, i.e. conclude that the treatment in question is effective. Theoretically, this could mean that acupuncture is a miracle cure which is useful for every single condition in every single setting. But sadly, there are no miracle cures. Therefore, something is likely to be badly and worryingly amiss. We[38] and others[39] have shown that Chinese trials of acupuncture hardly ever produce a negative finding. In other words, one does not need to read the paper, one already knows that it is positive—even more extreme: one does not need to conduct the study, one already knows the result before the research has started.

A recent systematic review[40] of all RCTs of acupuncture published in Chinese journals confirms these suspicions. A total of 840 RCTs were found. Among these, 838 studies (99.8%) reported positive results and only two trials (0.2%) reported negative findings. The authors concluded that *publication bias might be major issue in RCTs on acupuncture published in Chinese journals reported, which is related to high risk of bias*. High risk of bias in this context means 'too good to be true'.

4.9. The Role of Criticism

Criticism produces progress. Progress without criticism is almost unthinkable. Criticism is therefore important, whether we like it or not. Of course, I am not talking about criticism such as 'YOU ARE AN IDIOT'. In fact, that sort of thing is not criticism at all; it's an insult. I am also not thinking about criticism like 'YOUR ARGUMENT IS IDIOTIC'. In this chapter, I will focus on criticism that is constructive, well-argued and based on reasonably sound evidence.

Luckily, in medicine, we have plenty of this type of criticism. Its aim is to improve healthcare of the future for the

---

[38]   https://www.ncbi.nlm.nih.gov/pubmed/10406751.
[39]   https://www.ncbi.nlm.nih.gov/pubmed/9551280.
[40]   http://online.liebertpub.com/doi/pdfplus/10.1089/acm.2014.5346.abstract

benefit of us all. Most of the major medical journals are full of criticism, and many medical conferences are entirely or partly devoted to it. For instance, frequently cited papers in medicine's top journals regularly point out that:

- Too much of the current medical research is unreliable.
- Many conventional therapies are not based on good evidence (see section 2.5).
- Many treatments can cause severe adverse effects.
- Patients frequently do not get treated in a timely fashion.
- Modern medicine is too often inhumane.

The hope is that, by disclosing these and many other deficits, appropriate actions can be taken to improve the situation and make progress. But the process is hardly ever straight forward. All too often it is slow, inadequate and impeded by logistical and other obstacles. Therefore, it is crucial that constructive criticism continues to be encouraged. Many clinicians, researchers and other experts have dedicated their lives to this very task.

What I just described is the situation in conventional medicine. How about the role of criticism in SCAM? There is certainly not less to criticise in SCAM than in conventional medicine. So, are all the journals of SCAM full of criticism of SCAM? Are there regular conferences focused on criticism? Are SCAM practitioners keen to hear about the weaknesses of their beliefs, theories, practices, etc.? The short answer to all these questions is no!

Yet, SCAM advocates are by no means averse to voicing criticism. In fact, they criticise almost non-stop. But there is a fundamental difference: they criticise (often rightly) conventional medicine, and they criticise those (sometimes rightly) who criticise SCAM. When it comes to criticising their own practices, however, there is a deafening silence. The consequences of this situation are easy to see for everyone, and they can be dramatic:

- The SCAM journals publish nothing that could be perceived to be negative for the business of SCAM practitioners (see section 4.10).
- SCAM conferences rarely, if ever, schedule critical lectures.
- Self-critical thinking has remained an almost alien concept in SCAM.
- The very few people who dare to criticise aspects of SCAM from the 'inside' are ousted or declared to be incompetent or worse.
- Little action is taken to initiate change.
- The assumptions of SCAM remain unaltered for centuries.
- Progress is all but absent, and much of SCAM has degenerated into a cult.

These are, of course, stark conclusions. Let me therefore provide just three case histories exemplifying the notorious lack of criticism from three major SCAM disciplines: chiropractic, acupuncture and homeopathy.

Chiropractic

The chiropractic profession has been reminded time and time again that their claim to be able to effectively treat paediatric conditions is unsubstantiated. Yet chiropractors seem to remain in denial, famously documented by the British Chiropractic Association suing Simon Singh for libel after he disclosed that they 'happily promote bogus treatments' for children.[41]

Some chiropractors claim that, after this libel action, things have changed and that chiropractors are finally getting their act together. However, hundreds, if not thousands, of websites continue promoting chiropractic for childhood conditions. If things had really changed, one would expect that the chiropractic profession protests regularly, sharply and effectively to

---

[41] https://www.theguardian.com/commentisfree/2008/apr/19/controversi esinscience-health.

shame the charlatans amongst their midst. Crucially, one would expect the chiropractic professional organisations to oust their bogus members systematically and swiftly. Yet, the truth is that none of this seems to be happening.

On the contrary, books on chiropractic paediatrics, and periodicals like the *Journal of Pediatric, Maternal and Family Chiropractic*[42] remain popular and respected within the chiropractic profession. In other words, there is hardly any effective criticism from within the chiropractic profession to address this dangerous nonsense, and progress is therefore all but absent.

Acupuncture

Acupuncture Today is a popular online publication for people interested in acupuncture. On their website, we find an article which, in my view, is remarkable.[43] Here are some excerpts:

> A more efficient method for diagnosis and treatment by remote medical dowsing has been found and used in acupuncture with great success. The procedure involves a pendulum, a picture of the patient, an anatomy book, a steel pointer, and a very thin bamboo pointer…
>
> By dowsing the picture of the patient with the right hand and using a bamboo pointer to touch the lower head of the pterygoid muscle in the anatomy book with the left hand, it will be evident by the circular movement of the pendulum that these muscles now have good energy. This is done before the needle is inserted. In this manner all points can be checked for ailments such as TMJ, stroke, backaches, and neck and shoulder problems before needling. When the needles are placed and after the needling procedure, energy can be checked using the pendulum. By being very accurate on the location of acupuncture points, less treatments will be needed to obtain results. Another point is Small Intestine 19, a local point which is also very effective. Good results

---

[42]   http://chiropracticpediatrics.sharepoint.com/Pages/default.aspx.
[43]   http://www.acupuncturetoday.com/mpacms/at/article.php?id=31308.

are obtained by careful and accurate needling. Therefore, the number of visits are few…

Dowsing is a diagnostic aid that has been used for other situations and can be very helpful to acupuncturists. In conclusion, I feel that remote dowsing is a great approach to diagnosis and treatment.

I tried to find some acupuncturists who had objected to this nonsense, but I was not successful in my endeavour. The article was published years ago, yet, so far, no acupuncturist seems to have criticised it. I have also tried to see whether articles promoting such quackery are rare exceptions in the realm of acupuncture, or whether they are regular occurrences. My impression is that the latter seems to be the case. Criticism from acupuncturists of quackery promoted by fellow acupuncturists never seems to emerge.

Homeopathy

During the Liberian Ebola epidemic, a German homeopathic journal published the following interesting article[44] providing details about an international team of homeopaths that travelled to Liberia to cure Ebola patients. Here are a few excerpts (in my own translation):

In mid-October, an international team of 4 doctors travelled to the West African country for three weeks. The mission in a hospital in Ganta, a town with about 40,000 inhabitants on the border to Guinea, ended as planned on 7 November. The exercise was organised by the World Association of Homeopathic Doctors, the Liga Medicorum Homoeo-pathica Internationalis (LMHI), with support by the German Central Association of Homeopathic Doctors. The aim was to support the local doctors in the care of the population and, if possible, also to help in the fight against the Ebola epidemic. The costs for the three weeks' stay were

---

44   http://www.homoeopathie-online.info/homoeopathische-aerzte-helfen-in-liberia/.

financed mostly through donations from homeopathic doctors.

'We know that we were invited mainly as well-trained doctors to Liberia, and that or experience in homeopathy was asked for only as a secondary issue', stresses Cornelia Bajic, first chairperson of the DZVhA (German Central Association of Homeopathic Doctors). The doctors from India, USA, Switzerland and Germany were able to employ their expertise in several wards of the hospital, to help patients, and to support their Liberian colleagues. It was planned to use and document the homeopathic treatment of Ebola-patients as an adjunct to the WHO prescribed standard treatment. 'Our experience from the treatment of other epidemics in the history of medicine allows the conclusion that a homeopathic treatment might significantly reduce the mortality of Ebola patients', judges Bajic. The successful use of homeopathic remedies has been documented for example in Cholera, Diphtheria or Yellow Fever.

The news of this expedition made headlines across the world and most homeopaths would therefore have known about it. Many seemed impressed by the effort. I am, however, not aware of a single criticism from within the realm of homeopathy of the dangerous idea of treating Ebola homeopathically.

There are many more examples, but these three case histories must suffice. They support my impression that, in SCAM, criticism from the 'inside' is extremely rare. Consequently, progress is non-existent or painfully slow. And the consequence of that is, of course, that patients treated by SCAM practitioners tend to receive medical care that is obsolete.

Chapter 5

Healthcare Practitioners

Cured yesterday of my disease, I died last night of my physician. — Matthew Prior

5.1. The Tricks of the SCAM Trade

Considering its many flaws, the current popularity of SCAM might come as a surprise. Practitioners of SCAM claim that it is due to SCAM's effectiveness and safety. As there is precious little data to support this assumption,[1] it cannot be the true explanation. Could it be due to consumers being systematically misled? Over the years, I got the impression that there are certain 'tricks of the trade' which SCAM practitioners tend to employ in order to convince the often all too gullible public of the value of their services.

Treating non-existing conditions

There is nothing better for the SCAM business than to treat a condition that the patient does not actually have. Many SCAM practitioners have made a true cult of this ploy. Go to a chiropractor and you will probably receive a diagnosis of 'subluxation'. See a TCM practitioner and you might be diagnosed as suffering from 'chi deficiency' or 'chi blockage'. Each branch of

---

[1]   https://www.hive.co.uk/Product/Edzard-Ernst/Oxford-Handbook-of-Complementary-Medicine/16450051.

SCAM has its own diagnoses. They differ greatly but have one thing in common: they are figments of the SCAM practitioner's imagination.

The beauty of a non-existing diagnosis is, of course, that the practitioner can treat it, and treat it, and treat it... until the client either runs out of money, patience or both. Shortly before this occurs, the practitioner can proudly announce to his patient, 'you are now healthy'. This happens to be true, of course, because the patient has been fine all along.

Maintenance treatment

Another 'trick of the trade' is to persuade the patient of the necessity of 'maintenance' treatment. This term describes the regular treatment of an individual who is entirely healthy but who, according to the SCAM practitioner, needs regular treatments in order not to fall ill in future. Many chiropractors, for instance, claim that maintenance treatment is necessary for keeping a person's spine aligned—and only a well-serviced spine will keep all our body's systems working perfectly. It is like with a car, they claim: if you don't service it regularly, it will sooner or later break down. To many 'worried well' consumers, this might sound convincing. However, the efficacy of maintenance treatment is more than doubtful,[2] yet the benefits to the chiropractor's bank account cannot be doubted.

Things must get worse before they get better

Many patients fail to experience an improvement of their condition or might even feel worse after receiving SCAM. Practitioners tend to tell these patients that this is entirely normal because things have to get worse before they can get better. They often call this a 'healing crisis', a phenomenon for which no compelling evidence exists. Imagine a patient with moderately severe symptoms—say back pain—consulting a

---

[2]   https://www.ncbi.nlm.nih.gov/pubmed/19465044.

SCAM practitioner and receiving treatment. There are only three things that can happen to her:

- she can get better,
- she might experience no change at all,
- or she might get worse.

In the first scenario, the practitioner would obviously claim that his therapy is responsible for the improvement. In the second scenario, he might say that, without his therapy, things would have deteriorated. In the third scenario, he would tell his patient that the healing crisis is the reason for her experience. In other words, the myth of the healing crisis is a ploy to prevent even patients who do not benefit from SCAM from stopping their contributions to the practitioner's cash-flow.

A cure takes a long time

Imagine a patient—let's again assume she suffers from back pain—who, even after several SCAM sessions, has not improved. In this situation, most people would stop having (and paying for) the treatment. And this is, of course, a serious threat to the practitioner's income. Luckily, there is a 'trick of the trade' to minimise the risk: the SCAM practitioner explains that the patient's condition has been going on for a very long time (if this is not the case, the practitioner would explain that the symptom might be relatively recent but the underlying condition is chronic). This means, the SCAM practitioner would then explain, that a cure will also have to take a very long time—after all, Rome was not built in one day! This plea to carry on with the SCAM despite any the lack of improvement of symptoms is not justifiable on medical grounds. It is, however, entirely justifiable based on financial needs of the SCAM practitioners.

The problem is due to conventional medicine

A further 'trick of the trade' is the notion that a patient's problems are due to the poisonous drugs prescribed by her doctor. SCAM thrives on conspiracy theories (see section 3.4), and the one of the evil 'medical mafia' is an all-time favourite. It enables SCAM practitioners to instil a good dose of fear into the minds of their patients, a fear that minimises the risk of them returning to real medicine (see section 3.2).

Detox

The logical consequence of this poisoning scenario is that patients urgently need to 'detox'. As it happens, SCAM is, according to SCAM practitioners, ideally suited to achieve this aim. Detox is short for detoxification which, in real medicine, is the term used for weaning addicts off their drugs. In SCAM, it is used as a marketing slogan.

- The poisons in question are never accurately defined. Instead, we hear only vague terminologies such as metabolic waste products or environmental toxins. The reason is simple: once the poison is named, we would be able to measure it and test the efficacy of the treatment in question in eliminating it from the body. But this is the last thing SCAM practitioners want because it would soon establish how bogus their claims are.
- None of the SCAMs claimed to detox our bodies eliminates any toxin (unless, of course, we consider cash to be a poisonous substance).
- Our body has powerful organs and mechanisms to detoxify (skin, lungs, kidneys, liver). These take care of most of the toxins we are exposed to. If any of these organs fail, we do not require SCAM; in this case, we are more likely to need an A&E department's intensive care.

The test of time

Many SCAMs have been around for hundreds, if not thousands of years. To the enthusiasts, this signals that they have 'stood the test of time'. Practitioners of SCAM tell us that the age of their therapy is like a badge of approval from millions of people, a badge that surely weighs more that modern scientific studies.

Would anyone argue that, because a hot-air balloon is an older technology than an aeroplane, it is better suited for transporting people? The fact that acupuncture was developed thousands of years ago might just mean that it was invented by relatively ignorant people who understood too little about the human body to create a truly effective intervention. And the fact that blood-letting was used for centuries (and thus killed millions) might teach us a lesson about the true value of 'the test of time' in medicine.

Natural is good

People working in advertising would confirm that the label 'natural' is a great boost for sales of all sorts of things. Practitioners of SCAM have long appreciated this fact and exploited it to the best of their abilities. But think again:

- There is nothing natural in thrusting a patient's spine beyond the physiological range of motion (as in chiropractic).
- There is nothing natural in endlessly diluting and shaking remedies which may or may not have their origin in a natural substance (homeopathy).
- There is nothing natural in sticking needles into the skin of patients (acupuncture).

Moreover, the notion of a benign 'mother nature' is naïvely misleading. Ask someone who has been at sea during a storm or who has been struck by lightning.

Energy

Energy is a popular term in SCAM. Yet, SCAM providers do not really mean energy when they use the word; they mean 'vital force' or one of the many related terms. They use 'energy' because this sounds modern and impressive to many consumers. Crucially, it avoids disclosing how deeply steeped the therapists are in vitalism and vitalistic ideas. While rational thinkers have discarded such concepts more than a century ago, SCAM practitioners have retained it—mainly, I fear, because it is good for business.

Stimulating the immune system

'Your immune system needs stimulating!' This trick of the trade is almost obligatory in SCAM. Conventional clinicians might try to stimulate the immune system in certain, rare circumstances. More often they need to achieve the opposite effect and use powerful drugs to suppress the immune system. But even when they aim at stimulating a patient's immune system, they would not use any form of SCAM because:

1. The 'immune stimulants' of SCAM do not really stimulate the immune system.
2. Stimulating a normal immune system is hardly possible.
3. For many of us, stimulating the immune system would not be desirable.

But, in SCAM, the ploy of stimulating the immune system has proven to attract consumers and is therefore an effective way to keep the cash flowing.

Conclusions

There are many tricks of the SCAM trade misguiding us to attribute value to SCAM. Their main aims seem to be:

- to attract gullible consumers,
- to improve the SCAM practitioner's cash-flow.

5.2. Inside the Brain of a Scam Practitioner

Is the mind of the typical SCAM proponent different from that of a rational person? Adrian Furnham, a UK professor of psychology, has looked at this question in some detail. One of his investigations[3] concluded that *older people, with more modern*

---

3   https://www.ncbi.nlm.nih.gov/pubmed/19878620.

health worries, and who believe in the paranormal are more likely to believe that complementary and alternative medicine works, possibly because of a more intuitive, 'holistic', thinking style. In another study,[4] he concluded that *concern about health, belief about modern medicine and complementary/alternative medicine are logically interrelated. Those who have high modern health worries tend to be more sceptical about modern medicine and more convinced of the possible role of psychological factors in personal health and illness.* And in a third investigation,[5] he showed that *patients consult different practitioners, general or alternative, on the basis of a combination of their level of skepticism about orthodox medicine, their life-style, and other health beliefs.*

I have often felt that SCAM enthusiasts prefer belief to logic and emotions to reason. An obvious sign for the lack of rational thinking is the abundance of fallacies used to defend SCAM. One of many personal anecdotes might explain what I mean: recently, I was interrupted during a lecture by my host who felt this was the right moment for voicing her opinion. In my talk, I had shown evidence that, contrary to common belief, the use of homeopathy is not free of risks. My host's argument was as typical as it was fallacious. She angrily stated that conventional medicines cause much more serious side effects than homeopathics, and therefore homeopathy has its value. This argument is popular with SCAM enthusiasts, but it is based on a classical fallacy [Box 12].

Even the most abominable safety record of conventional medicine would be no reason to tolerate the deficiencies of SCAM. Moreover, comparisons of the risks of SCAM with those of conventional treatments are always misleading. Of course, aromatherapy, reflexology, homeopathy, etc. have fewer side effects than chemotherapy, by-pass surgery or bone marrow transplants. The true value of any therapy is not determined by its risks alone, but by the balance between the risks and the benefits. As homeopathics generate no benefits beyond

---

4   https://www.ncbi.nlm.nih.gov/pubmed/17456283.
5   https://www.ncbi.nlm.nih.gov/pubmed/9395630.

a placebo effect, a risk/benefit comparison between homeo-pathy and any evidence-based therapy cannot ever favour homeopathy.

Box 12
Explanations of the 'tu quoque' fallacy

- The deplorable number of deaths on the road does not justify unsafe trains.
- Aeroplane accidents are no support for the concept of flying carpets.
- You neighbour beating up his wife does not entitle you to be nasty to your spouse.
- Your suspicion that everyone is cheating is no justification to be dis-honest yourself.
- The high fatality rate of one hospital is not a justification for negligence in another institution.

Another example is the 'post hoc, ergo propter hoc' fallacy. It is firmly ingrained into the minds of SCAM enthusiasts. If a patient receives a treatment and subsequently gets better, what could be more tempting than to assume that the treatment was the cause of the improvement? This conclusion seems as obvious as it can be erroneous. Apart from the treatment *per se*, a range of phenomena exists that can cause or contribute to improvement: the placebo effect, the natural history of the ill-ness, the regression towards the mean and so on (see section 2.1). In other words, patients do frequently get better after administering useless remedies.

'Absence of evidence is not evidence of absence of effect.' This *bon mot* is much-liked by SCAM proponents. If, for a given SCAM, we have no good evidence for its effectiveness, we cannot assume that it is ineffective, they claim. The principle is, of course, entirely correct. We have not identified life on other planets, for instance, but we cannot be sure that no extra-terrestrial life exists. However, the conclusion SCAM propo-nents draw from this principle is seriously misleading. They argue that it is reasonable to use unproven treatments until the day when evidence emerges that proves it to be ineffective. In healthcare, it is unwise, dangerous and unethical to give the benefit of the doubt to under-researched therapies. In the interest of our patients, we are obliged to use treatments that are supported by sound evidence for effectiveness, while those that do not fall into this category should be avoided.

The more I discussed with SCAM enthusiasts over the last years, the more I had to realise that their logic is often fallacious. To see such fallacious thinking in action, we need not look far. The internet is rife with SCAM articles making ample use of it. The 'HOMEOPATHY HUB', for instance, lists seven points in defence of homeopathy[6] which provide us with an intriguing insight into the mind of homeopaths.

1. There are many types of evidence that should be considered when evaluating the effectiveness of a therapy. These include scientific studies, patient feedback and the clinical experience of doctors who have trained in a CAM discipline.

2. Many conventional therapies and drugs have inconclusive evidence or prove to be useful in only some cases, for example SSRIs (anti-depressants). Inconsistent evidence is often the result of the complexity of both the medical condition being treated and the therapy being used. It is not indicative of a therapy that doesn't work.

3. Removing all therapies or interventions that have inconsistent or inconclusive evidence would seriously limit the public and the medical profession's ability to help treat and ease patients suffering.

4. All over the world there are doctors, nurses, midwives, vets and other healthcare professionals who integrate CAM therapies into their daily practice because they see effectiveness. They would not use these therapies if they did not see their patients benefitting from them. For example in the UK, within the NHS hospital setting, outcome studies demonstrate effectiveness of homeopathy.

5. Practitioners of many CAM therapies belong to registering bodies which expect their members to comply to the

---

6   http://www.4homeopathy.org/2017/05/05/charity-commission-consultation-ends-19th-may/.

highest professional standards in regards to training and practice.

6. In the UK the producers and suppliers of CAM treatments (homeopathy, herbal medicine etc.) are strictly regulated.

7. As well as providing valuable information to the growing number of people seeking to use CAM as part of their healthcare, CAM charities frequently fund treatment for those people, particularly the elderly and those on a low income, whose health has benefitted from these therapies but who cannot afford them. This meets the charity's criterion of providing a public benefit.

Even a minimal amount of critical analysis discloses these seven arguments as misleading and fallacious:

1. 'Patient feedback and the clinical experience of doctors' are not evidence of therapeutic effectiveness (see section 2.1).

2. Yes, the evidence for conventional medicine is often inconclusive; therefore, we need to rely on proper assessments of the totality of the reliable data. If that fails to be positive (as is the case for homeopathy and several other forms of SCAM), we are well advised not to employ the treatment in question in routine healthcare but use a therapy that is well-supported by sound evidence (see above).

3. Removing all treatments for which the best evidence fails to be positive — such as homeopathy — would greatly improve healthcare and reduce cost; it is one of the aims of evidence-based medicine (EBM).

4. Yes, some healthcare professionals do employ useless therapies. They perhaps need to be educated in the principles of EBM. Outcome studies have normally no control groups and therefore are not adequate tools for testing the effectiveness of medical interventions (see section 2.1).

5. The highest professional standards regarding training and practice of nonsense will still result in nonsense.

6. The proper regulation of nonsense can only generate proper nonsense.
7. Yes, SCAM charities frequently fund bogus treatments, and this is a deplorable waste which ought to be stopped.

If we assumed that only lay-practitioners have adopted this type of illogical thinking, we would be wrong. Sadly, medical school does not seem to convey an absolute protection from fallacious arguments. A British GP, for instance, recently published an article[7] which gives an intriguing insight into the mind of a medically trained SCAM practitioner (the references in square brackets were added by me, and refer to my brief comments below):

...Homeopathy can be helpful for pretty much any condition [1], whether as the main treatment [1], as a complement to a conventional treatment [2] to speed up the healing process [1], or to lessen the side-effects of a pharmacological medication [1]. It can be helpful in the treatment of emotional problems [1], physical problems [1] and for multi-morbidity patients [1]. I find it an invaluable tool in my GP's toolbox and regularly see the benefits of homeopathy in the patients I treat [3]...

There are many conditions for which I have found homeopathy to be effective [1]... There are, however, a multitude of symptomatic treatments available to suppress symptoms, both on prescription and over-the-counter. Most symptoms experienced by patients in this context result from the body's attempt to eliminate the infection. Our immune systems have spent thousands of years refining this response; therefore it seems counter-intuitive to suppress it [4].

For these types of acute conditions homeopathy can work with the body to support it [1]. For instance, homeopathic

---

7   https://www.hippocraticpost.com/integrative/homeopathy-general-practice/.

Arsenicum album (arsenic) is a classic remedy for diarrhoea and vomiting that can be taken alongside essential oral rehydration [1]. And in influenza I've found Eupatorium perfoliatum (ague or feverwort) to be very helpful if the patient is suffering with bony pain [3].

...Unless it is clinically imperative for a pharmacological intervention, I will always consider homeopathy first [5] and have successfully prescribed the homeopathic remedy Nux vomica (strychnine) for women suffering from morning sickness [5]. Problems associated with breastfeeding such as mastitis have also responded well to the classic remedies Belladonna (deadly nightshade) and Phytolacca (pokeweed), while I have found Urtica urens (dog nettle) effective in switching off the milk supply to prevent engorgement when the mother stops breastfeeding [3].

..."Heart sink" patients are clearly suffering from pain and discomfort, which is blighting their lives. This is understandably frustrating for them, for they know full well something is awry but there is no medical evidence for this... Homeopathy affords me another approach in trying to help these patients [1,3]. It doesn't work for them all, but I'm frequently surprised at how many it does help [3].

The beauty of homeopathy is that it combines mental and emotional symptoms with physical symptoms [3]. When the right remedy is found it appears to stimulate the body to recognise how it is being dysfunctional and corrects this, with no suppression, just a correction of the underlying disturbance [3]. Thus homeopathy not only eliminates unwanted symptoms [1], it dramatically improves a patient's overall well-being [1].

...Homeopathy... enables me to reduce the number of painkillers and other drugs I'm prescribing [1,3]. This is particularly true for older multi-morbidity, polypharmacy patients [1] who are often taking huge amounts of medication.

Contrary to what most homeopaths will tell you, I believe homeopathic treatment does have side-effects — positive side-effects! [1] It fosters an enhanced doctor patient relationship [1]. The process of eliciting the relevant information to select a remedy enables me to better understand the patient's condition and helps me to get to know them better [3]. And the patient, seeing that the doctor is interested in the idiosyncrasies and detail of their disease, finds themselves heard and understood [3]. In short, since training in homeopathy I enjoy my job as a GP and my relationship with patients so much more [3].

1. This statement is not supported by good evidence; on the contrary, in 2017, the European Academies Science Advisory Council issued a statement that confirmed many other independent verdicts: ...*we agree with previous extensive evaluations concluding that there are no known diseases for which there is robust, reproducible evidence that homeopathy is effective beyond the placebo effect...*[8]
2. The founding father of homeopathy, Samuel Hahnemann, was vehemently against combining homeopathy with other treatments and called clinicians who disregarded this order 'traitors'.[9]
3. This is a statement of belief, absent any sound evidence.
4. This assumption is simply wrong.
5. This would be ethically questionable; patients have a right to be treated with the most effective treatments available, and homeopathy is not amongst them.

5.3. Little SCAM and Big Pharma

One thing that unites most SCAM proponents is their intense dislike for 'Big Pharma'. Essentially, they see this sector as:

---

[8]   http://www.easac.eu/fileadmin/PDF_s/reports_statements/EASAC_Homepathy_statement_web_final.pdf.
[9]   https://www.hive.co.uk/Product/Professor-Edzard-Ernst/Homeopathy--The-Undiluted-Facts--Including-a-Comprehensive-A-Z-Lexicon/19719982.

- Driven purely by profit.
- Employing unethical means to maximise profit.
- Not caring for the needs of patients.
- Attacking SCAM for fear of losing profit.

And, of course, they claim that 'Little SCAM', is fundamentally different from 'Big Pharma'.

I have no intention of defending the pharmaceutical industry. Pharmaceutical companies are usually responsible to their share-holders and that constellation can lead to excesses which are counter-productive to our needs, to put it mildly. However, the notion that Little SCAM is fundamentally different deserves some scrutiny.

In SCAM, there are certainly not as many mega-enterprises as in the pharmaceutical industry, but nobody can deny that many sizeable SCAM firms exist which make sizeable profits. And what about those parts of SCAM that are not into selling any products at all? Think of acupuncture, for instance. Well, SCAM therapists are not exempt from the need to make a living. Sure, this is on a different scale from the millions made by Big Pharma, but it undeniably constitutes a need to make a profit. If we multiply the relatively small sums involved by the vast number of therapists who practise today, the grand total of Little SCAM might even approach a similar order of magnitude as that of Big Pharma.

And what about those unethical means of Big Pharma for securing or maximising profits? During my many years of involvement in Little SCAM, I have witnessed several incidents which I would not hesitate to call unethical. One of the least pleasant, from my point of view, was the discovery that several German homeopathic manufacturers had given large sums of money to a 'journalist' who used these funds to systematically defame me.[10]

---

[10] http://www.quackometer.net/blog/2012/07/german-homeopathy-companies-pay-journalist-who-smears-uk-academic.html.

And what about the charge that Big Pharma does not care for the suffering patient? Little SCAM would never do that! Sadly, this is a myth too. As discussed repeatedly in this book, SCAM practitioners, their organisations and their supporters make a plethora of therapeutic claims which are not substantiated by good evidence. Who could deny that misleading patients into making wrong and damaging healthcare decisions is not the opposite of 'caring'? What seems even worse, in my view, is the behaviour that might follow the exposure of false claims. If someone is courageous enough to disclose the irresponsibility of bogus claims, he might be attacked or even taken to court by those who have done wrong.[11]

And then there is the notion of Big Pharma trying to suppress Little SCAM. I call this a myth too—at least I have never seen a jot of evidence for the assumption. Even those who circulate the rumour cannot, when challenged, produce any evidence. Also, don't we all know how many of the big pharmaceutical firms buy into the SCAM market as soon as they see a commercially viable opportunity? Does that look like suppression?

Big Pharma is also regularly accused of scientific misconduct (section 4.6). It can occur in different guises:

- drawing conclusions which are not supported by the data,
- designing studies such that they will inevitably generate a favourable result,
- cherry-picking the evidence,
- hiding unfavourable findings,
- publishing favourable results multiple times,
- submitting data-sets to multiple statistical tests until a positive result emerges,

---

[11]   http://edzardernst.com/2012/10/chiropractic-lessons-that-have-not-been-learnt/.

- defaming scientists who publish unfavourable findings,
- bribing experts,
- prettifying or falsifying data.

Most of these despicable ploys are well-known to pseudo-scientists in all fields of inquiry. To pretend they are unknown in SCAM would be naïve. In addition to these 'time-tested' ways of committing scientific misconduct, SCAM proponents have innovated a few novel methods to distract from unwelcome truths. Here I offer you five of the ones currently used by Little SCAM.

The 'fatal flaw' method

Whenever a major trial fails to confirm the wishful thinking of SCAM proponents, the question arises: what can be done about yet another piece of unfavourable evidence? The easiest solution would be to ignore it, of course — and this is precisely what is often tried. But this tactic can never fully eliminate the unwanted evidence. It would be preferable to have a tool which invalidates the unwelcome study once and for all.

The 'fatal flaw' method is an attempt to achieve this goal by claiming that such studies have a 'fatal flaw' in the way the SCAM therapy was applied. As only the experts in the 'very special' SCAM can judge the adequacy of their therapy, nobody must doubt their verdict.

Acupuncture, for instance, is an ancient 'art' which only the very best of us will ever master — at least that is what we are being told. So, all Little SCAM needs to do about a negative study is to read the methods section of the published paper and authoritatively affirm that the way acupuncture was applied in this particular trial was inadequate. The wrong points were stimulated, or the right points were stimulated but not long enough (or too long), or the needling was too deep (or too shallow), or the type of needles employed were wrong, or the contra-indications were not observed etc. etc.

As nobody can tell a correct acupuncture from an incorrect one, this 'fatal flaw' method is fool-proof. Acupuncture fans need not study hard to find the 'fatal flaw', they only have to look at the result of a study: if it was favourable, the treatment was obviously done optimally by highly experienced experts; if the result was unfavourable, the therapists clearly must have been amateurs who picked up their acupuncture skills in a single weekend course. A reason for such judgements can always be found or, if all else fails, invented.

The outcome of the 'fatal flaw' method is most satisfactory and can be applied to all forms of SCAM — homeopathy, herbal medicine, reflexology, Reiki healing, colonic irrigation — you name it; the method works for all of them!

The non-conclusive method

The efficacy and effectiveness of medical interventions is best tested in clinical trials. The principle of a clinical trial is simple: typically, a group of patients is divided (preferably at random) into two subgroups, one is treated with the experimental treatment and the other (the 'control' group) with another option (often a placebo), and the eventual outcomes of the two groups is compared. If done well, such studies can tell us whether an outcome was caused by the intervention *per se* or by some other factor such as the natural history of the disease, regression towards the mean, etc. (see also section 2.1).

A clinical trial is a research tool for testing hypotheses; strictly speaking, it tests the 'null hypothesis': 'the experimental treatment generates the same outcome as the treatment of the control group'. If the trial shows no difference between the outcomes of the two groups, the null hypothesis is confirmed. In this case, we commonly speak of a negative result. If the experimental treatment was better than the control treatment, the null hypothesis is rejected, and we commonly speak of a positive result. Thus, clinical trials can only generate positive or negative results, because the null hypothesis is either confirmed or rejected — there are no grey tones between the black of a negative and the white of a positive study.

For SCAM enthusiasts, this creates a dilemma, particularly if lots of studies with negative results exist. In this case, the totality of the available trial evidence is negative which means the treatment in question cannot be characterised as effective. However, such an overall conclusion is unacceptable to SCAM proponents. Consequently, they look for ways to avoid this scenario.

One obvious way of achieving this aim is to re-categorise the results. What, if we invented a new category? What, if we called some of the negative studies by a different name? What about 'non-conclusive'? This way, we might end up with a situation where the majority of the evidence is, after all, positive. And this, of course, would give the impression that our ineffective treatment in question is effective!

The way to achieve this aim is to continue to call positive studies POSITIVE; we then call studies where the experimental treatment generated worse results than the control treatment (usually a placebo) NEGATIVE; and finally, we call those studies where the experimental treatment created outcomes which were not different from placebo NON-CONCLUSIVE.

In SCAM, this 'non-conclusive' method is well-established. For instance, the UK 'Faculty of Homeopathy' claim that *up to the end of 2011, there have been 164 peer-reviewed papers reporting randomised controlled trials (RCTs) in homeopathy. This represents research in 89 different medical conditions. Of those 164 RCT papers, 71 (43%) were positive, 9 (6%) negative and 80 (49%) non-conclusive.*[12]

This message was, of course, warmly received by homeopaths. The 'British Homeopathic Association', like many other organisations and individuals with an axe to grind, promptly repeated it: *The body of evidence that exists shows that much more investigation is required – 43% of all the randomised controlled trials carried out have been positive, 6% negative and 49% inconclusive.*[13]

Let's be clear what has happened here: the true percentage figures seem to show that 43% of studies (mostly of poor quality) suggest a positive result for homeopathy, while 57% of

---

[12]   http://facultyofhomeopathy.org/research/.
[13]   https://www.britishhomeopathic.org/#.

them (on average the ones of better quality) are negative. In other words, the majority of this body of evidence is negative. If we conducted a proper systematic review, we would, of course, need to account for the quality of each study. In this case, we would have to conclude that homeopathy is not supported by sound evidence. The application of the 'non-conclusive' method has thus turned this overall result upside down: black has become white! No wonder that it is so popular with proponents of SCAM!

The phony review method

Systematic reviews are widely considered to be the most reliable type of evidence for judging the effectiveness of therapeutic interventions (see section 2.1). They should be focused on a well-defined research question and identify, critically appraise and synthesise the totality of the high-quality research relevant to the specific research question.

One strength of systematic review is that they minimise selection and random biases by considering all the evidence of a predefined nature and quality. A crucial precondition, however, is that the quality of the primary studies is critically assessed. If this is done adequately, the researchers will usually be able to determine how robust any given result is, and whether high-quality trials generate similar findings as those of lower quality. If there is a discrepancy between findings from rigorous and flimsy studies, it is advisable to trust the former and discard the latter when forming a final verdict.

And this is where systematic reviews of SCAM often run into difficulties. For any given research question, we usually have a paucity of primary studies. Equally important is the fact that many of the available trials tend to be of low or very low quality. Consequently, there often is a lack of reliable studies, and this makes it all the more important to include a robust, critical evaluation of the primary data. Not doing so would render the overall result of the review less than reliable — in fact, such a paper would not qualify as a systematic review at all; it would be a phony review, i.e. a review which pretends to be systematic but, in fact, is not. Such papers are a menace in that they can seriously mislead us.

This is precisely where some promoters of SCAM seem to see their opportunity for making their unproven therapy look as though it was evidence-based. Phony reviews can be manipulated to yield a desired outcome. Unless we bother to do a considerable amount of research, we are highly unlikely to notice that anything is amiss. All the SCAM proponent needs to do is to smuggle the phony review past the peer-review process — hardly a difficult task, given the plethora of SCAM journals (see section 4.10) with editors bending over backwards to publish almost any rubbish as long as it promotes SCAM.

A prime example of a phony review is a 'systematic' review commissioned by the UK General Chiropractic Council after the chiropractic profession got into trouble after suing Simon Singh for libel.[14] The review was a thinly disguised attempt to show that, at least for some conditions, chiropractic was effective. Its lengthy conclusions seemed complex but encouraging:

> Spinal manipulation/mobilization is effective in adults for: acute, subacute, and chronic low back pain; migraine and cervicogenic headache; cervicogenic dizziness; manipulation/mobilization is effective for several extremity joint conditions; and thoracic manipulation/mobilization is effective for acute/subacute neck pain. The evidence is inconclusive for cervical manipulation/mobilization alone for neck pain of any duration, and for manipulation/mobilization for mid back pain, sciatica, tension-type headache, coccydynia, temporomandibular joint disorders, fibromyalgia, premenstrual syndrome, and pneumonia in older adults. Spinal manipulation is not effective for asthma and dysmenorrhea when compared to sham manipulation, or for Stage 1 hypertension when added to an

---

[14] https://www.theguardian.com/science/2010/apr/15/simon-singh-libel-case-dropped.

antihypertensive diet. In children, the evidence is inconclusive regarding the effectiveness for otitis media and enuresis, and it is not effective for infantile colic and asthma when compared to sham manipulation. Massage is effective in adults for chronic low back pain and chronic neck pain. The evidence is inconclusive for knee osteoarthritis, fibromyalgia, myofascial pain syndrome, migraine headache, and premenstrual syndrome. In children, the evidence is inconclusive for asthma and infantile colic.

Chiropractors across the world were relieved, and to the present day cite this paper as evidence that chiropractic has at least some evidence base. What they omit to tell us is the fact that the review authors:

- failed to formulate a focused research question,
- invented their own categories of inconclusive findings (see above),
- included studies which had little to do with chiropractic,
- failed to assess the quality of the included primary studies included in their review.

If, for a certain condition, three trials were included, for instance, two of which were positive but of poor quality and one was negative but of good quality, the authors would conclude that, overall, there is sound evidence. Thus, the phony review method is a simple way to turn shoddy evidence into something respectable.

The non-evidence method

My systematic review[15] of the available RCTs of chiropractic for asthma showed quite clearly that the best evidence suggested chiropractic was ineffective for that condition. But chiropractors did not like to hear that, therefore they conducted

---

[15]   https://www.ncbi.nlm.nih.gov/pubmed/19373624.

another systematic review[16] which concluded that chiropractic is an effective therapy for asthma: *...the eight retrieved studies indicated that chiropractic care showed improvements in subjective measures and, to a lesser degree objective measures...*

How can this be? The second review included all sorts of papers, even case reports and surveys, which are not evidence at all (see section 2.1). In fact, proponents of SCAM regularly succeed in smuggling non-evidence into such reviews to confirm their wishful thinking. The case of chiropractic for asthma does by no means stand alone, but is merely one example of how we are being misled by non-evidence masquerading as evidence.

The EBM method

The most widely used definition[17] of evidence-based medicine (EBM) is probably this one: *The judicious use of the best current available scientific research in making decisions about the care of patients. Evidence-based medicine (EBM) is intended to integrate clinical expertise with the research evidence and patient values.* David Sackett's own definition[18] is a little different: *Evidence based medicine is the conscientious, explicit, and judicious use of current best evidence in making decisions about the care of individual patients. The practice of evidence based medicine means integrating individual clinical expertise with the best available external clinical evidence from systematic research.*

Even though the principles of EBM are now widely accepted, there are those who point out that EBM has its limitations[19] [Box 13].

---

[16]   https://www.ncbi.nlm.nih.gov/pubmed/20195423.
[17]   http://www.medicinenet.com/script/main/art.asp?articlekey=33300.
[18]   http://www.bmj.com/content/312/7023/71.
[19]   https://www.ncbi.nlm.nih.gov/pubmed/15036077.

Box 13
The main criticisms of EBM

- Reliance on empiricism,
- Narrow definition of evidence,
- Lack of evidence of efficacy,
- Limited usefulness for individual patients,
- Threat to the autonomy of the doctor/patient relationship.

Advocates of SCAM have long been keen to point out that EBM is not applicable to their area. They tend to refer directly to the definitions of EBM and argue that EBM must fulfil at least three criteria:

1. external best evidence,
2. clinical expertise and
3. patient values or preferences.

Next, they try to convince us that almost everything in SCAM is evidence-based. Let me explain this with two deliberately extreme examples.

Crystal therapy for curing cancer

There is not a single trial for crystal healing. But crystal therapists might nevertheless claim that some cancer patients respond favourably to their treatment. Thus the 'best' available evidence is clearly positive, they could argue. Certainly, the clinical expertise of these crystal therapists is positive. So, if a cancer patient wants crystal therapy, all three preconditions are fulfilled and crystal therapy is entirely evidence-based.

Chiropractic for asthma

As mentioned above, the best evidence available to date does not demonstrate the effectiveness of chiropractic for asthma. But never mind, the clinical expertise of chiropractors may well be positive. If the patient also has a preference for chiropractic, at least two of the three conditions are fulfilled. Therefore — on balance — chiropractic for asthma is (almost) evidence-based.

The 'EBM method', as applied by many SCAM practitioners, is thus a ploy for turning the principles of EBM upside down. Its application leads us straight back into the dark ages of medicine when anything was legitimate as long as some charlatan could convince his patients to endure his quackery and pay for it — if necessary with his life.

5.4. Holistic Dentistry

Holistic dentistry is being promoted on virtually thousands of websites. But what is it? This article[20] tries to explain:

> ...holistic dentistry involves an awareness of dental care as it relates to the entire person, with the belief that patients should be provided with information to make choices to enhance their personal health and wellness...
> Some of the philosophies include:
> — Alternatives to amalgam/mercury fillings
> — Knowing and following proper mercury removal
> — Multi-disciplinary, or integrated, health care
> — Nutritional and preventive therapies and temporomandibular joint disorder therapy.

To me, this sounds like a string of platitudes designed to lure in new customers and boost business:

- An awareness that the mouth and its content is part of the whole body is not a philosophy but a banality.
- Providing information to patients is an ethical and legal duty for all dentists.
- Alternatives to amalgam have existed for decades and are used by all dentists.
- Integrated health is a most questionable fad (see section 5.2).
- Nutrition is part of conventional healthcare.
- Temporomandibular joint disorders are an issue for conventional dentistry.

---

[20]   http://circleofdocs.com/beyond-the-teeth-holistic-dentistry-examines-the-body-as-a-whole/.

But perhaps another article might do a better job at explaining what 'holistic dentistry' is all about:[21]

> ...Holistic dentistry is not considered a specialty of the dental profession, but a philosophy of practice. For those dentists who take the concept to its core, holistic dentistry includes an understanding of each patient's total well-being, from their specific cosmetic, structural, functional, and health-related dental needs to the concerns of their total body and its wellness. Holistic dentists tend to attract very health-conscious individuals.
>
> Some of the things holistic dentists are especially concerned about are the mercury found in traditional amalgam dental fillings, fluoride in drinking water, and the potential relationship of root canal therapy to disease in other parts of the body. Holistic dentists' primary focus is on the underlying reasons why a person has dental concerns, and then help correct those issues by strategic changes in diet, hygiene and lifestyle habits.
>
> Natural remedies to prevent and arrest decay and periodontal (gum) disease can also be utilized. Many holistic dentists are skilled in advanced levels of nutritional physiology and use natural means of healing patients, often avoiding the more standard use of systemic antibiotics, pain control management and surgical procedures.

This partly describes what good dentists have always done, and partly it is pure nonsense. For instance, natural remedies for tooth decay and gum disease? Which remedies precisely? I know of not one that is backed by sound evidence.

The more I read about holistic dentistry, the more I suspect that it is a smokescreen for smuggling bogus treatments into conventional dentistry, a bonanza of nonsense to attract gullible customers, a distraction for hijacking a few core principles from real dentistry, and a con for maximising the income of some dentists. 'Holistic dentistry', I fear, makes no

---

[21]   http://www.thehealthjournals.com/holistic-dentistry-means/.

more sense than holistic banking, holistic hairdressing, holistic pedicure, holistic carpentry, etc. Depending on the skill of the professional, dentistry, medicine, hairdressing, etc. are either good, not so good, or bad. The term holistic as it is currently used in dentistry is little more than a sales gimmick — much like in the rest of healthcare (section 3.3), I am afraid.

5.5. Doctors of Integrative Medicine

When physicians practise SCAM, they often call it 'integrative' or 'integrated' medicine (IM). We therefore need to ask, what exactly is IM? There are several definitions, and it seems that, over the years, IM fans have been busy moving the definitional goal posts quite a bit. The original principle of IM was that it incorporates 'THE BEST OF BOTH WORLDS', but this idea has subsequently been modified considerably.

- IM is a *comprehensive, primary care system that emphasizes wellness and healing of the whole person…*[22]
- IM *views patients as whole people with minds and spirits as well as bodies and includes these dimensions into diagnosis and treatment.*[23]

The UK 'College of Medicine and Integrated Health' once offered the most fascinating definition of them all:

- *IM is a holistic, evidence-based approach which makes intelligent use of all available therapeutic choices to achieve optimal health and resilience for our patients.*[24]

This sentence oozes political correctness and might therefore impress some people. But, on closer scrutiny, it turns out to be more than a little odd. Let's take the content of this definition step by step:

---

[22]   https://www.ncbi.nlm.nih.gov/pubmed/?term=Arch+Intern+Med.+2002%3B162%3A133-140.
[23]   https://www.ncbi.nlm.nih.gov/pubmed/11159553.
[24]   http://www.bathgped.co.uk/website/IGP318/files/Building%20Resilience%20for%20the%20Healthy%20Heart.pdf.

1) IM is holistic

Holism has always been at the core of any type of good health-care (see section 3.3). To state that IM is holistic misleads people into believing that conventional medicine is not holistic. It also implies that medicine might become more holistic through the addition of SCAM. Yet I cannot imagine anything less holistic than diagnosing patients by merely looking at their iris (iridology) or assuming all disease stems from subluxations of the spine (chiropractic), for example. In a nutshell: the holistic argument is a straw-man, if there ever was one.

2) IM is evidence-based

This statement is pure wishful thinking. If we look what is being offered in IM clinics, we find an endless array of treatments that are not supported by good evidence, as well as many for which the evidence is simply negative.

Even on the academic level, IM is far removed from evidence. In 2012, I published an analysis of the '3rd European Congress of Integrated Medicine' which had taken place in 2010 in Berlin.[25]. For this purpose, I read all the 222 abstracts and categorised them according to their contents. The results showed that the majority was on unproven SCAMs and none related to conventional treatments (a fact that seems to contradict the notion that 'integrated' means the use of interventions from both 'worlds').

The 2016, International Congress on Integrative Medicine & Health[26] provided me with the opportunity to check whether this situation has since changed. There were around 400 abstracts, and I did essentially the same type of analysis as before, except this time I also assessed whether the conclusions of each paper were positive (expressing something favourable about the subject at hand), negative (expressing something negative about the subject at hand) or neither of the two. On

---

25   http://onlinelibrary.wiley.com/doi/10.1111/j.1365-2796.2011.02417.x/
      abstract.
26   http://online.liebertpub.com/doi/full/10.1089/ACM.2016.29003.abstracts.

this occasion, mind–body therapies proved to be the most popular subject with 49 papers, followed by acupuncture (44), herbal medicine (37), integrative medicine (36), chiropractic and other manual therapies (26), TCM (19), methodological issues (16), animal and other pre-clinical investigations (15) and tai chi (5). The rest of the abstracts were on a diverse array of other subjects. Again, not a single paper related to a conventional therapy. None of these papers discussed IM and its assumptions critically. The analysis according to the direction of the conclusions showed that 260 papers were positive, 5 negative and the rest was equivocal.

Essentially, my two analyses show that IM is not about evidence-based treatments. It is almost exclusively about SCAMs that are unproven or disproven.

3) IM is intelligent

It is hard to take this claim seriously. Is the implication here that conventional medicine is not intelligent? Could this be another straw-man?

4) IM uses all available therapeutic choices

This element of the definition seems to give 'carte blanche' to IM proponents for employing anything they like. Do they seriously believe that patients should have ALL AVAILABLE treatments? Do they not know that much of what is available is rubbish and that responsible healthcare is about applying the most effective therapies for any condition at hand?

5) IM aims at achieving optimal health

This must be the third straw-man; it implies that conventional healthcare professionals do not aim to restore their patients to optimal health. Surely, achieving optimal health of their patients is the aim of any clinician.

In view of all this, the following 7 conclusions about IM seem justified, in my view:

1. Proponents of IM tend to mislead us with nonsensical terminology and definitions.
2. IM promotes two main principles: a) the use of SCAM and b) holism.
3. Holism is at the heart of all good medicine; IM is at best an unnecessary distraction from it.
4. Using holism to promote SCAM seems counter-productive (see section 3.3).
5. The integration of unproven and disproven treatments must render healthcare not better but worse.
6. IM therefore flies in the face of common sense and medical ethics.
7. IM is a disservice to patients.[27]

The last point is exemplified by IM doctors' attitudes towards immunisations, for example. A 2017 study[28] evaluated the attitudes and practices regarding vaccination of the 1,419 members of the American Board of Integrative and Holistic Medicine. The survey assessed their use of and confidence in vaccination recommendations. Its findings showed that IM physicians are less likely to administer vaccinations than physicians practising conventional medicine. Among the 44% who did provide vaccinations, 35% used alternative schedules regularly. IM physicians were also more likely to accept a connection between vaccinations and autism or other chronic diseases. Physicians practising IM therefore tend to endanger public health by their non-evidence-based attitudes towards vaccination.

5.6. The German 'Heilpraktiker'

Because of the extraordinary freedom of practice, official status and public acceptance, the German 'Heilpraktiker' (literally translated: healing practitioner) is the envy of SCAM

---

[27]   https://www.ncbi.nlm.nih.gov/pubmed/15065622.
[28]   https://www.ncbi.nlm.nih.gov/pubmed/28160764.

practitioners the world over. This profession is perhaps best understood by its fascinating history.[29]

When the Nazis came to power in 1933, German healthcare was dominated by lay practitioners who were organised in multiple organisations. The Nazis felt the need to reorganise this situation to bring it under their control. *To re-unify German medicine under the banner of 'Neue Deutsche Heilkunde', the Nazi officials created the 'Heilpraktiker' – a profession which was meant to become extinct within one generation. The 'flag ship' of the 'Neue Deutsche Heilkunde' was the 'Rudolf Hess Krankenhaus' in Dresden. It represented a full integration of CAM and orthodox medicine. An example of systematic research into CAM is the Nazi government's project to validate homoeopathy. Even though the data are now lost, the results of this research seem to have been negative. Even though there are some striking similarities between today's CAM and yesterday's 'Neue Deutsche Heilkunde' there are important differences. Most importantly, perhaps, today's CAM is concerned with the welfare of the individual, whereas the 'Neue Deutsche Heilkunde' was aimed at ensuring the dominance of the Aryan race.*[30]

The Nazis thus offered to grant all SCAM practitioners official recognition by establishing them under the newly created umbrella of 'Heilpraktiker'. At the same time, they needed to please the powerful lobby of conventional doctors and therefore decreed that the 'Heilpraktiker' was barred from educating a second generation of this profession. Therefore, the Heilpraktiker was destined to become extinct within decades. The Nazi rulers clearly hoped that SCAM would soon become an established part of 'Neue Deutsche Heilkunde' (New German Medicine). However, for a range of reasons, this never happened.

After the war, the Heilpraktiker profession went to court and won the right to educate their own students. Today, they are a profession that uses all sorts of SCAMs. The German Heilpraktiker has no mandatory medical training; a simple test

---

29   https://www.ncbi.nlm.nih.gov/pubmed/9157042.
30   https://www.ncbi.nlm.nih.gov/pubmed/11264971.

to show that they know the legal limits of their profession suffices for receiving an almost unrestricted licence for practising medicine.

> ...the "Heilpraktiker" is allowed to practice medicine, like medically trained physicians... Anybody 25 years old or older, with a secondary school certificate, and free of disease can participate in a test, conducted by the local health authorities to 'exclude danger to the health of the nation.' In the case of failure, this test can be repeated ad libitum. Having passed this test, the heilpraktiker is allowed to practice the whole realm of medicine, except for gynecology, dentistry, prescription of medication, and healing infectious diseases... Although several cases of fatal errors in treatment are known, the greatest risk in the heilpraktiker's practice is the omission of proper diagnostics and therapies, which is risk by omission...[31]

Unsurprisingly, there are numerous reports of Heilpraktikers doing harm to their patients.[32] However, because there is no effective post-marketing surveillance system in this area, the frequency of harm is essentially unknown. Because of the risk to public health, a group of experts has recently published a document to stimulate a constructive discussion about the German Heilpraktiker.[33] Essentially, we suggested that the Heilpraktiker has introduced two hugely different quality standards into the German healthcare system. In the interest of the patient and of good healthcare, this danger must be addressed. We therefore demanded that the profession of the Heilpraktiker is either completely abolished or reformed such that it no longer poses a threat to public health in Germany.

---

[31] https://www.ncbi.nlm.nih.gov/pubmed/20084355.
[32] http://edzardernst.com/2016/08/fatalities-in-a-german-alternative-medicine-clinic-caused-by-3bp/.
[33] https://www.aerzteblatt.de/down.asp?id=19264.

5.7. Veterinarians

In the mid-1810s, Samuel Hahnemann, the founder of homeopathy, gave a lecture about homeopathy for animals. Ever since, homeopathy has been used in veterinary medicine. Initially, veterinary medical schools took a dim view of homoeopathy, and the number of veterinary homeopaths remained small. Today, however, veterinary homeopathy has become increasingly popular. In some countries, veterinary homeopaths have their own professional organisations, while in other countries veterinarians are banned from practising homeopathy.

What diseases do homeopathic veterinarians treat? One article[34] informs us that the *conditions frequently treated are: arthritis, lameness, cruciate rupture, chronic diarrhoea, atopy, allergy, autoimmune disorders (auto-immune), periodic ophthalmia (moon blindness, recurrent uveitis, recurrent ophthalmia, ERU), head shaking (head-shaking), hip dysplasia, COPD, sweet itch, laminitis, corneal ulcer, elbow dysplasia, RAO, DJD, OCD, bone cysts, pasteurellosis (pasteurella), chlamydia, cryptosporidia, pneumonia, meningitis, mastitis, ringworm, epilepsy, pyoderma, eczema, dermatitis, eosinophilic myositis, eosinophilic granuloma, rodent ulcer, miliary eczema (miliary dermatitis), kidney problems, liver problems (hepatopathy), cystitis.*

This, of course, begs the question whether homeopathy is effective for any of these conditions. A systematic review[35] included 18 RCTs which were disparate in nature, representing four species and eleven different medical conditions. Reliable evidence, free from vested interest, was identified in only two trials:

- One suggested that a homeopathic preparation of Coli bacteria had a prophylactic effect on porcine diarrhoea.

---

[34]   http://www.veterinary-homeopathy.co.uk/homeopathy.html.
[35]   https://www.ncbi.nlm.nih.gov/pubmed/25324413.

- The other one demonstrated that individualised homeopathic treatment did not have a more beneficial effect on bovine mastitis than placebo intervention.

The authors conclusions are clear: *Mixed findings from the only two placebo-controlled RCTs that had suitably reliable evidence precluded generalisable conclusions about the efficacy of any particular homeopathic medicine or the impact of individualised homeopathic intervention on any given medical condition in animals.*

A more recent systematic review[36] specifically assessed the efficacy of homeopathy in cattle, pigs and poultry. A total of 52 trials were included of which 28 trials were in favour of homeopathy, whereas 22 showed no medicinal effect. Cure rates for the treatments with antibiotics, homeopathy or placebo varied to a high degree, while the remedy used did not seem to make a significant difference. No study had been repeated under comparable conditions. The authors concluded that the use of homeopathy is unproven.

A further systematic review[37] evaluated the effectiveness of non-antimicrobials for mastitis in cows. Only studies comparing the treatment under investigation to a negative or positive control, or both, were included. Outcomes were clinical and bacteriological cure rates and milk production. A total of 39 articles corresponding to 41 studies were included. No evidence-based recommendations could be given for the use of an alternative or non-antimicrobial conventional treatment for mastitis. The authors concluded that *homeopathic treatments are not efficient for management of clinical mastitis.*

These conclusions are in line with several new trials that were not included in any of the above reviews. For instance, a study[38] tested the efficacy of homeopathic treatment in bovine clinical mastitis and concluded that *the results indicated no additional effect of homeopathic treatment compared with placebo.*

---

[36] http://veterinaryrecord.bmj.com/content/early/2016/12/09/vr.103779.full.
[37] https://www.ncbi.nlm.nih.gov/pubmed/28755947.
[38] https://www.ncbi.nlm.nih.gov/pubmed/28342609.

And a double-blind, placebo-controlled randomised trial[39] aimed at testing the efficacy of individualised homeopathy in the treatment of feline hyperthyroidism concluded that *the results of this study failed to provide any evidence of the efficacy of homeopathic treatment of feline hyperthyroidism.*

Most importantly, the conclusions are also in line with a recent statement of the European Academies Science Advisory Council.[40] This independent body of experts assessed the relevant evidence and concluded that *there is no rigorous evidence to substantiate the use of homeopathy in veterinary medicine and it is particularly worrying when such products are used in preference to evidence-based medicinal products to treat livestock infections.*

Despite this overwhelmingly negative evidence the Veterinary Dean of the UK Faculty of Homeopathy published this statement in 2017:[41]

> Homeopathy has a long history of being used successfully in veterinary practice for both domestic and farm animals. The EU recommends its use in its regulations on organic farms and is funding research into veterinary homeopathy as a way of reducing antibiotic use in livestock. It is nonsense to suggest that responsible pet owners and farmers are unable to distinguish between effective and ineffective medicines; they continue to use homeopathy because they see its benefits.

Other forms of SCAM used in veterinary medicine include chiropractic. This article[42] explains:

> ...Animal chiropractic (veterinary spinal manipulative therapy) focuses on the preservation and health/wellness

---

[39]　https://www.ncbi.nlm.nih.gov/pubmed/28077754.

[40]　http://www.easac.eu/fileadmin/PDF_s/reports_statements/EASAC_Ho mepathy_statement_web_final.pdf.

[41]　http://facultyofhomeopathy.org/response-to-petition-calling-on-the-rcvs-to-ban-homeopathy/.

[42]　http://www.observertoday.com/life/2017/05/veterinary-spinal-manipulative-therapy-animal-chiropractic/.

of the neuro-musculo-skeletal system. Chiropractic is the science that is centered around the relationship between the spine and the nervous system. The spine is your body's foundation and the nervous system, including your brain, spinal cord and nerves, controls your entire body. They must work together harmoniously to improve one's general health and their ability to heal. If the systems are not functioning to their highest potential you may experience changes in digestion, heart and lung function, reproduction and most evidently musculature. When adjacent joints are in an abnormal position, called a subluxation, the nervous system and all that it controls will be negatively impacted. If these subluxations are not corrected, they can result in prolonged inappropriate stimulation of nerves. This could result in reduced function internally, musculo-skeletal dysfunction and pain.

Spinal manipulation is the art of restoring full and pain free range of motion to joints and can greatly benefit an animal after they have experienced subluxations. The veterinarian will use their hands to palpate joints both statically and in motion. By doing this, they can determine where the animal is experiencing decreased motion or misaligned joints. Once identified, an adjustment can be performed. An adjustment or spinal manipulation is a gentle, specific, quick and low force thrust that will be applied at an angle specific to the different areas of motion in the spine and extremities. Only a certified animal chiropractor will understand the complexity involved in adjustments and can best assess if an animal can benefit from chiropractic care.

Many animals can benefit from this alternative therapy. If you notice that your animal has a particularly sensitive spot somewhere on their body, is walking or trotting differently and or not performing to the same ability they have previously, they may be a candidate for a chiropractic assessment. However, an animal does not need to be sick or injured to benefit from chiropractic care. Animals in good health or ones used for sporting activities are also prime candidates for chiropractic care. By maintaining your pet's proper spinal alignment and mobility they will attain optimal function of muscles, nerves and tissues that support the joints. When the body can move freely your pet will experience improved mobility, stance and flexibility, which can evolve into improved agility, endurance and overall performance. Finally, many people have never considered that chiropractic care can also benefit their animal by boosting their immune response. It can aid in providing a healthier metabolism and a vibrant nervous system which all facilitate your animal's natural ability to heal themselves from within. Chiropractic care can enhance the quality of your pet's life ensuring many active and healthy years to come.

But does animal chiropractic work? I failed to locate a single study or review to suggest that chiropractic is effective for specific conditions of animals.

Even acupuncture is increasingly being used for animals. An article of the Acupuncture Now Foundation,[43] for instance, claimed that *veterinary acupuncture is used successfully in many different animals...* How reliable is this statement? The only systematic review[44] in this area happens to be by my team and it concluded that *there is no compelling evidence to recommend or reject acupuncture for any condition in domestic animals. Some encouraging data do exist that warrant further investigation in independent rigorous trials.*

Thus, the evidence for veterinary SCAM is even less convincing than that in humans. Many therapies have never been tested, and those that have been submitted to trials have not been shown to be effective.

---

[43] https://acupuncturenowfoundation.org/doctors/putting-acupuncture-research-into-perspective/.
[44] https://www.ncbi.nlm.nih.gov/pubmed/16734078.

5.8. Nurses

In 2012, researchers from Aberdeen, UK, conducted a survey[45] to establish the use of SCAM by registered nurses, as well as their knowledge-base and attitudes towards it. They sent a questionnaire to 621 nurses and achieved a remarkable response rate of 86%. Eighty per cent of the responders admitted employing SCAM and 41% were using it currently. Only five nurses believed that SCAM was not effective and 74% would recommend it to others.

A similar review of nurses' attitudes towards SCAM concluded that *some nurses promote complementary therapies as an opportunity to personalise care and practice in a humanistic way. Yet, nurses have very limited education in this field and a lack of professional frameworks to assist them. The nursing profession needs to consider how to address current deficiencies in meeting the growing use of complementary therapies by patients.*[46]

A 2015 review[47] investigated nurses' knowledge of and attitudes towards SCAM, as well as their ability to communicate the risks and benefits of these therapies to patients. The researchers found that 66% of nurses had positive attitudes towards SCAM; while 77% did not possess a comprehensive understanding of the associated risks and benefits. The authors concluded that *the lack of knowledge about complementary and alternative medicine among nurses is a cause for concern, particularly in light of its widespread application.*

I think that the currently widespread acceptance of SCAM by nurses begs two important questions:

1. Why does the 'endeavour to improve the quality of care available to patients' require the use of SCAM?
2. Why are nurses not more concerned about the lack of evidence that underpins their use of SCAM?

---

[45]   https://www.ncbi.nlm.nih.gov/pubmed/22875353.
[46]   https://www.ncbi.nlm.nih.gov/pubmed/28167377.
[47]   https://www.ncbi.nlm.nih.gov/pubmed/25727902.

It is perhaps not all that difficult to comprehend why many nurses feel attracted by SCAM; if nothing else, it offers the opportunity to exercise compassion and empathy in patient care—and these are qualities that are often badly needed in conventional nursing. But it would be important (not just for nurses but for all healthcare professionals) to realise that compassion must be paired with evidence-based care and effective treatments rather than with the use of unproven and disproven therapies.

Therapeutic Touch (TT) is a SCAM typically used by nurses. A recent survey[48] showed that such treatments are incredibly popular: over 50% of the families that were asked admitted using them for children suffering from cancer. TT is said to channel 'healing energy' into the body of the patient which, in turn, is thought to stimulate the patient's self-healing potential. Proponents of TT claim that it is effective for a very wide range of conditions.

Most of the research into TT is badly flawed and its findings are therefore unreliable. A laudable exception is this recent clinical study[49] aimed at determining whether TT is efficacious in decreasing pain in preterm neonates. Fifty-five infants participated in this randomised clinical trial. Immediately before and after a painful heel lance procedure, nurses performed non-tactile TT with the infant behind curtains. In the sham condition, the therapist stood by the incubator without performing TT. The results showed no group differences in pain or any other outcome measure. The authors concluded that *Therapeutic Touch given immediately before and after heel lance has no comforting effect in preterm neonates. Other effective strategies involving actual touch should be considered.* These results are in line with those of a Cochrane review[50] which concluded that *there is no robust evidence that TT promotes healing of acute wounds.*

---

[48]   https://www.ncbi.nlm.nih.gov/pubmed/24307910.
[49]   https://www.ncbi.nlm.nih.gov/pubmed/23817594.
[50]   https://www.ncbi.nlm.nih.gov/pubmed/22696330.

Why then is TT specifically so popular with nurses? Part of the answer is that *New Age spiritualism has co-opted some of the language of physics, including the language of quantum mechanics, in its quest to make ancient metaphysics sound like respectable science. The New Age preaches enhancing your vital energy, tapping into the subtle energy of the universe, or manipulating your biofield so that you can be happy, fulfilled, successful, and lovable, and so life can be meaningful, significant, and endless. The New Age promises you the power to heal the sick and create reality according to your will, as if you were a god.*[51]

Another SCAM for nurses is the Bowen Technique, a SCAM that involves gentle rolling motions along the muscles, tendons and fascia. The therapy's distinctive features are the minimal nature of the physical intervention and pauses incorporated in the treatment. Proponents claim these pauses allow the body to 'reset' itself.

> Come along for ten-minute taster sessions and experience the Bowen Technique. It is appropriate for a wide range of acute and chronic conditions, including back pain, sciatica, neck, shoulder and knee problems, arthritis, asthma, migraine, sports injuries and stress. Ten-minute taster sessions will be offered so that you can experience the therapy first hand. Many find their aches and pains melt away![52]

With these words, the UK Royal College of Nursing advertised a course of Bowen Technique during their annual conference in 2017. Such advertisements fly in the face of science. In 2015, the Department of Health of Australia published the results of a review in which Bowen Technique was noted as one of 17 therapies for which no good evidence of effectiveness was found.[53] In fact, there is currently not a single trial testing the efficacy of Bowen Technique for any disease or symptom.

[51] http://www.skepdic.com/tt.html.
[52] https://www.rcn.org.uk/congress/agenda/bowen-therapy-sunday.
[53] https://en.wikipedia.org/wiki/Bowen_technique.

Essentially, all of this suggests that many nurses have adopted SCAM uncritically without asking whether there is sufficient evidence that this behaviour generates more good than harm. As so often in the realm of SCAM, the loser is bound to be the patient.

5.9. Midwives

A 2014 survey[54] monitored the use of SCAM by Scottish healthcare professionals involved in the care of pregnant women. A total of 135 professionals (midwives, obstetricians, anaesthetists) filled the questionnaire. A third of the respondents had prescribed or advised the use of SCAMs to pregnant women. The most frequently recommended modalities were: vitamins and minerals (55%); massage (53%); homeopathy (50%); acupuncture (32%); yoga (32%); reflexology (26%); aromatherapy (24%); and herbal medicine (21%). Midwives who had been in post for more than five years were the most likely group to recommend SCAM. The authors concluded that *despite the lack of safety or efficacy data, a wide variety of SCAM therapies are recommended to pregnant women by approximately a third of healthcare professionals.*

This high level of SCAM-usage by midwives is confirmed by two independent systematic reviews. The first[55] included all surveys assessing SCAM-use by midwives worldwide. Its findings suggest that most midwives recommend and employ SCAM. In some instances, the usage was close to 100%. Much of this practice was not supported by sound evidence for efficacy and some of the SCAMs had the potential to put patients at risk. The second review[56] concluded that *there is considerable support by midwives for the use of SCAM by expectant women. Despite this enthusiasm, currently there are few educational opportunities and only limited research evidence regarding SCAM use in midwifery practice. These shortfalls need to be addressed by the*

---

54   https://www.ncbi.nlm.nih.gov/pubmed/24512627.
55   https://www.ncbi.nlm.nih.gov/pubmed/22015222.
56   http://www.sciencedirect.com/science/article/pii/S1871519210000880.

profession. Midwives are encouraged to have an open dialogue with childbearing women, to document use and to base any advice on the best available evidence. The last point here seems crucial: for most SCAMs, the evidence is either absent, inconclusive or negative. Midwives advising their patients to try SCAM regardless of this fact are arguably not adhering to best practice and perhaps even violating ethical or legal standards.

Despite these concerns, the SCAM-use of midwifes is currently being promoted via the internet, books and newspapers. An example is an article in the UK *Guardian*[57] stating that *every woman needing pain relief while giving birth at University College London hospital (UCLH) is offered acupuncture, with around half of the hospital's midwives specially trained to give the treatment.*

Outside the UK, the situation is similar. A review[58] analysing the use of homeopathic prescriptions that are reimbursed by the French national health insurance during the period July 2011–June 2012 showed that a total of 120,110 healthcare professionals prescribed at least one homeopathic drug or preparation. They represented 43.5% of the overall population, nearly 95% of general practitioners, dermatologists and paediatricians, and 75% of midwives.

Numerous charities try to inform—often misinform—the public about SCAM (see also section 6.1). One example is a UK charity called 'Homeopathy Without Borders' (HWB).[59] This organisation promotes the use of homeopathic remedies worldwide, particularly in disaster-stricken and extremely deprived areas. The activities of HWB in 2013 included training midwives to administer and recommend homeopathic remedies: *We plan to initiate a training program in 2013 for Haitian midwives and birth attendants for homeopathic therapeutics in pregnancy, delivery and postpartum care.*

---

[57]   https://www.theguardian.com/healthcare-network/2015/oct/13/
       acupuncture-used-more-widely-nhs#comment-61323025.
[58]   https://www.ncbi.nlm.nih.gov/pubmed/25921648.
[59]   https://www.hwbna.org/.

All of this demonstrates that, like nurses, midwives seem to have adopted SCAM on a big scale and without questioning whether this behaviour is evidence-based or not.

5.10. Pharmacists

Pharmacists are frequently the only healthcare professional who consumers consult before trying a SCAM product. Therefore, it would be crucial that their recommendations are responsible and based on sound evidence. As a pharmacist, you must:

- Make patients your first concern.
- Use your professional judgement in the interests of patients and the public.
- Show respect for others.
- Encourage patients and the public to participate in decisions about their care.
- Develop your professional knowledge and competence.
- Be honest and trustworthy.
- Take responsibility for your working practices.

These seven principles were laid down by the UK General Pharmaceutical Council.[60] Similar guidelines exist the world over. But do pharmacists really adhere to them when dealing with SCAM?

A recent survey[61] with 887 student pharmacists explored their views on SCAM. The results showed generally favourable attitudes towards SCAM. There were strong indications that most students agreed with the long-obsolete concepts of vitalism. When asked about specific SCAMs, many students revealed positive views even on the least plausible and least evidence-based modalities like homeopathy or Reiki.

---

[60] https://www.pharmacyregulation.org/.
[61] https://www.ncbi.nlm.nih.gov/pubmed/?term=Student+pharmacists+ hold+generally+favorable+views+of+CAM%2C.

Considering the attitudes of pharmacy students, we should
not be surprised to learn about the stance of established
pharmacists and their professional organisations. The Austrian
Society of Pharmacists, for instance, stated that it is their aim to
find *explanatory models for the mechanisms of action of
homeopathy.*[62] This organisation also recommends a homeopathic emergency kit[63] to consumers which includes the
following remedies, doses and indications:

Aconitum C 30; 2 x 5 Glob, first remedy in cases of fever
Allium cepa C 12; 3 x 5 Glob, hay-fever or cold
Anamirta cocculus LM 12; 2 x 5, travel sickness
Apis mellifica C 200; 2 x 5 Glob, insect bites
Arnica C 200; 1 x 5 Glob, injuries
Acidum arsenicosum C 12; 3–5 x 5, food poisoning
Atropa belladonna C 30; 2 x 5 Glob, high fever
Cephaelis ipecacuahna C 12; 2 x 5 Glob, nausea/vomiting
Coffea arabica C 12; 2 x 5 Glob, insomnia and restlessness
Euphrasia officinalis C 12; 3 x 5 Glob, eye problems
Ferrum phosphoricum C 12; 2 x 5 Glob, nose bleed
Lachesis muta C 30; 1 x 5 Glob, infected wounds
Lytta vesicatoria C 200; 1–2 x 5, burns
Matricaria chamomilla C 30; 1 x 3 Glob, toothache
Mercurius LM 12; 2 x 5 Glob ear ache, weakness
Pulsatilla LM 12; 2 x 5 Glob, ear ache, indigestion
Solanum dulcamara C 12; 3 x 5 Glob, cystitis
Strychnos nux vomica LM 12; 2 x 5 Glob, hangover
Rhus toxicodendron C 200; 2 x 5 Glob, rheumatic pain

A quick reminder: C 200 means that the original substance has
been diluted 1: 10000000000000000000000000000000000000000
0000000000000000000000000000000000000000000000000000000000
0000000000000000000000000000000000000000000000000000000000
0000000000000000000000000000000000000000000000000000000000

---

[62] http://www.homresearch.org/homresearch.
[63] http://www.homresearch.org/wordpress/wp-content/uploads/2013/04/
      20_notfallapotheke.pdf.

0000000000000000000000000000000000000000000000000000000000
0000000000000000000000000000000000000000000000000000000000
0000000000000000000000000000000000000000000000000000000000
00000000000000000000000!!!

In my view, pharmacists selling implausible, unproven or disproven remedies are in danger of:

- breaking the ethical code of their profession,
- putting profit before responsible healthcare,
- lending credibility to quackery,
- risking their reputation as responsible healthcare professionals,
- endangering the health of many of their customers.

The Chief Scientist of the UK Royal Pharmaceutical Society seems to agree when stating: *the public have a right to expect pharmacists and other health professionals to be open and honest about the effectiveness and limitations of treatments. Surely it is now the time for pharmacists to cast homeopathy from the shelves and focus on scientifically based treatments backed by clear clinical evidence.*[64]

If that is so, what could be pharmacists' motivations in selling disproven SCAMs like homeopathic remedies? One reason would be that they are convinced of their efficacy. Whenever I talk to pharmacists, I do not get the impression that this is the case. During their training, pharmacists learn facts about homeopathy which clearly do not support the notion of efficacy. Some pharmacists might nevertheless be convinced of the efficacy of homeopathic remedies, but they would obviously not be well informed and thus find themselves in conflict with their duty to practise according to the current best evidence. On reflection therefore, strong positive belief can probably be discarded as a prominent reason for pharmacists selling bogus medicines like homeopathic remedies.

---

[64] http://edzardernst.com/2015/06/remove-homeopathy-from-pharmacies-royal-pharmaceutical-society-chief-scientist-challenges-profession-to-act/.

Another possible explanation is the notion that because patients want such products, pharmacists must offer them. When considering this argument, the tension between the ethical duties as a healthcare professional and the commercial pressures of a shop-keeper becomes painfully obvious. For a shop-keeper, it may be perfectly acceptable to offer any product customers might want. For a healthcare professional, however, this is not necessarily true. The ethical codes of pharmacists make it perfectly clear that the sale of unproven or disproven medicines is not ethical. Therefore, this often-cited notion may well be what pharmacists feel, but it does not seem to be a valid excuse for selling bogus medicines.

A variation of this theme is the argument that, if patients were unable to buy homeopathic remedies, they would only obtain more harmful drugs. The assumption here is that it might be better to sell harmless homeopathic placebos to avoid the potentially serious side effects of real but non-indicated medicines. In my view, this argument is nonsensical: if no (drug) treatment is indicated, professionals have a duty to explain this fact to their patients. In healthcare, a smaller evil cannot easily be justified by avoiding a bigger one; on the contrary, we should always thrive for the optimal course of action, and if this means reassurance that no medical treatment is needed, so be it.

Pharmacists working in large chain pharmacies often claim that they have no influence whatsoever over the range of products on sale on their premises. This perception may well be true. But equally true is the fact that healthcare professionals cannot be forced to violate their code of ethics. If a chain insists on selling bogus medicines, it is up to individual pharmacists and their professional organisations to stand up against such unethical malpractice. In my view, the argument is therefore not convincing and certainly does not provide an excuse for not finding a long-term solution to the problem.

An all too obvious motivation for selling SCAM products is the fact that pharmacists earn money by doing so. There clearly is a potential conflict of interest here, whether pharmacists want to admit it or not.

Realising these problems, some pharmacists have become critical towards SCAM; some even dare to make fun of SCAMs such as homeopathy. A laudable example of this is a US pharmacist who published this comment:[65] *I have worked at a homeopathic manufacturing plant. Yes, there is always a starting material, however sometimes it can get really shady... My favorite story is this one: We needed to do a dilution of uranium 200X. Problem is, you can't get uranium (unless you're Doc Brown), so we went to Hanford (this was a looong time ago) carrying a vial of water. When we got there and did a tour (the plant manager knew what we were going to do), we took the vial and held it up against a glass wall that was as close as we could get to the cooling chamber. That became our '1X' dilution. We went back to our lab and diluted it to 200X, in ethanol. We had a lot left over, and because it's illegal in WA to dump large quantities of ethanol down the drain, we needed a disposal service. Unfortunately, when we tried to explain that it was a 200X dilution (and that there wasn't even a single atom of uranium in there to begin with), they still wouldn't take it, because it said 'uranium' on the label. So we took a shovel and buried in the back of the plant, and never told anyone.*

---

[65]   https://www.reddit.com/r/skeptic/comments/2hwbgx/question_does_anyone_know_if_companies_which_make/.

Chapter 6

Patients and Consumers

I'm so gullible.
I'm so damn gullible.
And I am so sick of me being gullible.
– Lana Turner

6.1. Patient Choice

Patients' *choices include more than just which GP or hospital to use.* *[Patients] also have choices about [their] treatment decisions...*[1] Statements like this about patient choice abound; often they come from politicians who have more ambition to win votes than to understand the complexity of the issues at hand. Consequently, consumers might be forgiven for assuming that patient choice means we are all encouraged to indulge in the therapy that happens to take our fancy, while society foots the bill. Certainly, proponents of SCAM are fond of the assumption that the principle of patient choice provides 'carte blanche' for everyone who so wishes to have homeopathy, Reiki, Bach Flower Remedies, crystal healing, or any other SCAM — paid for, of course, by the taxpayer.

The reality, however, is very different. Anyone who has tried to choose their hospital will know that this is, in fact, far from easy. Deciding what treatment one might want to employ

---

[1]   http://www.nhs.uk/nhsengland/pages/nhsengland.aspx.

for this or that condition is even less straightforward. Patient choice has become a slogan used to score points in public debates but which frequently turns out to be next to meaningless. Often, the illusion of patients being in control must serve as a poor substitute for truly calling the shots.

Imagine you have a serious condition, say cancer. After you have gotten over the shock of this diagnosis, you begin to research on the internet and consider your options. Should you have surgery or faith healing; chemotherapy or homeopathy; radiotherapy or detox? Or imagine a patient who is essentially healthy but feels that she is a little stressed and therefore wants regular tai chi lessons combined with some probiotics and herbal medicines.

When paid for by public funds, a patient's choice cannot be about choosing between an evidence-based option and an unrealistic one. It must be confined to treatments which have been shown to do more good than harm. Using our notoriously tight healthcare budgets for dubious treatments is not just unwise, it is nothing short of unethical. If, for a given condition, there happen to be ten different, equally effective and safe options, we may indeed have a choice. Alas, this is rarely the case. Often, there is just one effective treatment. In such instances, the only realistic choice is between accepting or rejecting it.

And anyway, how would consumers know that ten different treatments are equally effective and safe? After going on the internet and reading a bit about them, we might delude ourselves that we know. But, as we discussed previously, the internet can be a very dangerous tool; it would tell a cancer patient that homeopathy, for instance, can be used to treat cancer.[2] Very few patients have sufficient knowledge for differentiating bogus from responsible information and making complex therapeutic decisions. We usually need an expert to help us with our choices [Box 13]. In other words, we usually require

---

[2]   http://edzardernst.com/2016/04/homeopathy-for-cancer-not-again-no-no-no/.

our doctor to guide us through the jungle of false claims, unreliable promotion, proven benefits and potential risks.

BOX 14
Qualities a medical expert should possess

- Sufficient clinical experience.
- Good understanding of the patient's condition.
- Sound knowledge of evidence-based medicine.
- Ability to understand scientific papers.
- Skills of systematic analysis and critical thinking.

Once we accept this to be true, we arrive at a reasonable concept of what patient choice really means in relation to deciding between two or more treatments: the concept of shared decision making. And this is fundamentally different from the naïve view of SCAM enthusiasts promoting the idea that patient choice opens the door to opting for any SCAM paid for by society.

To be meaningful, choice needs to be responsible; to be responsible, it needs to be guided by sound evidence; to be guided by sound evidence, it usually needs the input of an impartial expert. If not, choice degenerates into arbitrariness, and healthcare deteriorates to something akin to Russian roulette. To claim, as some SCAM proponents do, that the principle of patient choice gives everyone the right to use unproven or disproven treatments at the expense of the taxpayer is pure nonsense based on little more than wishful thinking.

6.2. When Orthodox Medicine Has Nothing More to Offer

The notion that the use of an unproven or disproven therapy is justified in cases where, for a specific patient, conventional medicine has run out of options is heavily promoted by SCAM proponents. At first glance, it may seem both logical and ethical. According to this argument, SCAM should be employed for patients 'given up' by conventional doctors, even if the evidence fails to show that SCAM is effective. An article[3] entitled 'When Orthodox Medicine Has Nothing More to Offer' is a typical example for the reasoning that underpins the notion. The following sections are excerpts from it (the numbers in brackets were inserted by me and refer to my comments below):

> ...Some people come when conventional treatments can no longer offer them anything to save their lives. This is a frightening time for them and although the homeopathic approach may not offer a cure at this late stage of their illness [1] it can often offer hope of a different kind [2]. Sometimes it helps people to outlive the prognosis given to them by months or even years [3]. Sometimes it helps them need less in the way of conventional medicine including pain killers [4] and offers them continuing support despite progressive disease [5]...
>
> One wonderful aspect of the homeopathic approach is that it can be a very important opportunity to help someone re-evaluate their life and their health [5].
>
> Sometimes hurts in the past have never been healed and sitting with someone as they describe difficult experiences can be itself therapeutic [5]. Combining this therapeutic listening time with substances from nature that gently stimulate the body's own healing potential [4] can be an approach that through patient demand and research we can demonstrate is really worth offering to many more people...

1. The implication that homeopathy can cure cancer at an early stage is irresponsible and wrong.
2. One does not need a disproven treatment such as homeopathy[4] for offering hope to patients.

---

3   https://www.britishhomeopathic.org/charity/how-we-can-help/articles/womens-health/breast-cancer/.
4   http://www.easac.eu/fileadmin/PDF_s/reports_statements/EASAC_Homepathy_statement_web_final.pdf.

3. A medical prognosis never entails a precise time of
    death; it is based on statistics and therefore refers to a
    likelihood, not a certainty. Thus, it is normal and fre-
    quent that many patients outlive the average survival
    time of their condition.
4. There is no good evidence to suggest that this claim is
    correct.
5. In conventional medicine, patients with progressive
    disease also receive continuing support, for instance in
    hospice care.

This short excerpt shows how desperate patients are being
misled into making dramatically wrong choices. If a lay-person
reads the text (without my comments), it probably would seem
reasonable to her, particularly if she happens to be a vulnerable
and desperate cancer patient. Therefore, many people fall for
this type of misleading logic and end up thinking that
homeopathy or other disproven SCAMs are reasonable options
when orthodox medicine has nothing more to offer. But the
claim of SCAM practitioners that conventional healthcare has,
in certain cases, nothing to offer is quite simply not true:

- Supportive and palliative care are established and
  important parts of conventional medicine.
- The implied scenario where a patient is told by her
  oncology team: 'sorry but we cannot do anything else
  for you', does not occur in real life (if it ever happens
  to you, I advise changing oncologist immediately). In
  some cases, there may be no curative options left, but
  there is always a way to ease symptoms.

Thus, the argument 'when orthodox medicine has nothing
more to offer' turns out to be viciously misleading. And the
subsequent argument of some SCAM practitioners, 'as "they"
have given you up, we now offer you our effective treatments',
is equally wrong. For most SCAMs, there is no good evidence
to show that they work. In other words, one falsehood is added
to another falsehood—and sadly, two untruths do not make a
truth.

6.3. The Wellness Mania

There are few terms in the realm of SCAM that are more popular—and more abused—than 'wellness'. An entire industry has developed around it and has associated itself closely with integrative medicine (section 5.5): *Integrative medicine, also referred to as complementary and alternative medicine, provides a set of tools and philosophies intended to enhance wellness...*[5] But what precisely is wellness in SCAM? According to the 'National Wellness Institute':[6]

- Wellness is a conscious, self-directed and evolving process of achieving full potential.
- Wellness is multidimensional and holistic, encompassing lifestyle, mental and spiritual well-being, and the environment.
- Wellness is positive and affirming.

The authors of another article[7] explained in more detail: *While the concept of wellness is still evolving, it is generally recognized that wellness is a holistic concept best represented as a continuum, with sickness, premature death, disability, and reactive approaches to health on one side and high-level wellness, enhanced health, and proactive approaches to health and well-being on the other. It is further acknowledged that wellness is multidimensional and includes physiologic, psychological, social, ecologic, and economic dimensions. These multiple dimensions make wellness difficult to accurately assess as multiple subjective and objective measures are required to account for the different dimensions. Thus, the assessment of wellness in individuals may include a variety of factors, including assessment of physiologic functioning, anthropometry, happiness, depression, anxiety, mood, sleep, health symptoms, toxic load, neurocognitive function, socioeconomic status, social connectivity, and perceived self-efficacy.*

---

5   https://www.ncbi.nlm.nih.gov/pubmed/28595441.
6   http://www.nationalwellness.org/?page=Six_Dimensions.
7   http://online.liebertpub.com/doi/full/10.1089/ACM.2016.0268.

To me, this sounds vague and almost seems like yet another ploy aimed at separating gullible consumers from their hard-earned cash. Yes, there is lots of money to be made in the wellness business; for instance, with so-called 'wellness retreats'. Such places usually offer a wide range of SCAMs in luxurious holiday settings for the 'well to do'. Of course, there is nothing wrong with a luxuriously relaxing holiday. But wellness retreats often make concrete health claims, and it is therefore legitimate to ask whether these claims are backed up by evidence.

One of the few studies in this area assessed what effects a wellness-retreat experience might have on healthy volunteers. Outcomes were assessed on arrival and on departure as well as six weeks after the retreat. The wellness programme consisted of a *holistic, 1-week, residential, retreat experience that included many educational, therapeutic, and leisure activities and an organic, mostly plant-based diet.* Significant improvements were noted in almost all outcome measures after one week. Some of these improvements were sustained even after six weeks. There were, for instance, significant reductions in abdominal girth, weight and blood pressure. The authors concluded that *the retreat experiences can lead to substantial improvements in multiple dimensions of health and well-being that are maintained for 6 weeks.*

In my view, these conclusions are more promotional than scientific by nature. But what do the results of this study really indicate? They suggest that people who are enjoying a luxury holiday with regular exercise and a healthy diet will feel better, relax and lose weight. This is unsurprising and indisputably a good thing, but I fail to see what it has to do with 'wellness'.

The current wellness mania is exemplified by an article[8] offering five tips for finding a 'wellness chiropractor' (the numbers in brackets were added by me and refer to my comments below).

---

[8]   http://articles.mercola.com/sites/articles/archive/2016/02/28/wellness-chiropractic.aspx?x_cid=20160228_lead_wellness-chiropractic_twitterdoc.

Does the practice focus on vertebral subluxation [1] and wellness? Physical, biochemical, and psychological stress may result in spinal subluxations [1] that disrupt nerve function [2] and compromise your health [3]. If you're looking for a wellness chiropractor, it's essential that this be the focus. Some chiropractors confine their practice to the mechanical treatment of back and neck pain, and this is something you need to be aware of beforehand.

1. **Does the doctor 'walk the talk'?** If he or she is overweight, looks unhealthy, or does not live a healthy lifestyle, this speaks volumes regarding their commitment to wellness [4].

2. **Do the two of you 'click'?** Do you like each other? Do you communicate well? Avoid a doctor [5] who seems rushed, talks down to you, or seems disinterested in listening to your concerns [6].

3. **Does the doctor use objective assessments of nerve function?** Since your care is not based just on addressing pain, your chiropractor should be using some form of objective assessment of your nerve function, as spinal subluxations [1] can sometimes be asymptomatic [7]. Non-invasive instruments that measure the electrical activity in your muscles, and/or a thermal scanner [8] that evaluates the function of your autonomic nervous system can be used, for example.

4. **What treatment techniques are used?** Chiropractic techniques include low-force adjustments by hand, and more forceful adjustments using instruments [9]. Ask which technique would be used on you [10], and if you have a preference, make sure the doctor [5] is willing to use it.

1. 'Spinal subluxation' is a non-entity that has no place in rational healthcare; it is based on the wishful thinking of some chiropractors.[9]

---

[9]   https://www.ncbi.nlm.nih.gov/pubmed/16092955.

2. I am not aware of any evidence to suggest this to be true.
3. As subluxations do not exist, it seems safe to say that this is nothing but fantasy.
4. The assumption seems to be that only a healthy chiropractor is a good chiropractor.
5. Chiropractors are being promoted as doctors — good for generating a healthy income but misleading, in my view.
6. These are qualities that are required from everyone — your waiter, bus conductor, butcher, etc.
7. Non-existent entities are always asymptomatic.
8. A test with very poor reliability.
9. Misleading statement; manual 'adjustments' can also be forceful and are often more forceful than those using instruments.
10. This statement suggests that informed consent is not what chiropractic patients can automatically count on (see section 2.6).

An almost amusing example of 'wellness mania' is an article entitled *'Donald Trump is more holistic and more health orientated than Hilary Clinton'*,[10] where the reader is introduced to 'Donald Trump's Wellness Plan'.

…What has catapulted Trump to the top of GOP polls? His frank, honest — and admittedly blunt — discussion about illegal immigrants, many of whom he correctly noted were criminals: Rapists, murderers and gang thugs…

For one, 'The Donald'… is a consumer of organic food. His daughter, Ivanka, has said that the whole family consumes mostly fresh, organic meals which she often prepares herself.

In addition, Trump's children help oversee foods served at the family hotels — meals that include vegan, organic and

---

[10] http://www.naturalnews.com/050521_Donald_Trump_organic_lifestyles_healthy_living.html.

gluten-free in-room dining choices. And when it can, the hotel chain obtains locally-grown organic foods as a way of giving back to the communities they serve. The family's diet even has a name: The Trump Wellness Plan, which fits with Trump's overall health and fitness lifestyle…

…a known golf lover, Trump says it's an ideal way to diminish stress and ponder business tasks while walking. He says, 'I find it opens my mind to new possibilities, and I can problem-solve very effectively while I'm on the golf course.'

I think I can rest my case: wellness is one of the most abused terms in the realm of SCAM.

6.4. Value for Money

Fans of SCAM often target politicians with the argument that their treatments are excellent value, and politicians are often duly impressed. For instance, the UK Member of Parliament David Tredinnick stated publicly that *alternative treatments are incredibly good value for money*.[11] Commissioned by Prince Charles, the Smallwood Report of 2005 famously claimed that the UK National Health Service would save millions if GPs were to use more homeopathy. My public objection to the seriously flawed report might have prevented it being taken seriously by politicians, but sadly it also cost me my job (the full story can be read in my memoir).

For some enthusiasts, the notion that SCAM saves money is too tempting to resist—but is it true? To answer this question, we need reliable evidence, not potentially biased opinion. Fortunately, several good studies are now available. Researchers from Sheffield, for instance, published a systematic review of 14 economic evaluations of homeopathy.[12] They concluded that *although the identified evidence of the costs and potential benefits of homeopathy seemed promising, studies were highly heterogeneous and*

---

[11] https://en.wikipedia.org/wiki/David_Tredinnick_(politician).
[12] https://www.ncbi.nlm.nih.gov/pubmed/23397477.

had several methodological weaknesses. It is therefore not possible to draw firm conclusions based on existing economic evaluations of homeopathy.

There are, of course, distinct types of economic evaluations of medical interventions; the most basic of these simply compares the cost of one treatment with those of another. In such an analysis, SCAMs would normally win against conventional treatments, as they are generally inexpensive. If one, however, adds the treatment time into the equation, things become a little more complex; consultations in SCAM tend to be considerably longer than conventional ones, and if the therapist's time is costed, it is uncertain whether SCAM would still be cheaper. But even such evaluations would not provide very meaningful answers to most questions.

Much more relevant are cost–benefit analyses which compare the relative costs and outcomes of two or more treatments. Any cost–benefit analysis can only produce meaningfully positive results if the treatment in question is supported by sound evidence for effectiveness. A treatment that is not demonstrably effective cannot be cost-effective!

A recent study[13] took account of these issues and compared the healthcare costs for patients using additional homeopathic treatment (homeopathy group) with the costs for those receiving usual care (control group). Data from 44,550 patients were available for analysis. The total costs after 18 months were higher in the homeopathy group than in the control group with the largest differences between groups for productivity loss and outpatient care costs. Group differences decreased over time. For all diagnoses, costs were higher in the homeopathy group than in the control group. The authors concluded that, *compared with usual care, additional homeopathic treatment was associated with significantly higher costs. These analyses did not confirm previously observed cost savings resulting from the use of homeopathy in the health care system.* This study was recently extended, and the authors concluded that, *even when following-*

---

[13]   https://www.ncbi.nlm.nih.gov/pubmed/26230412.

up over 33 months, there were still cost differences between groups, with higher costs in the homeopathy group.[14]

What about chiropractic? Many chiropractors claim that their treatments save healthcare costs. Unfortunately, this assumption turns out to be less certain than they seem to believe. The aim of this systematic review[15] was to evaluate economic evaluations of chiropractic care compared to other commonly used approaches among adult patients with non-specific low back pain (LBP). Six RCTs and three full economic evaluations were included. The authors found similar effects for chiropractic and other types of care. Three low- to high-quality full economic evaluation studies compared chiropractic to medical care. Highly divergent conclusions were noted for economic evaluations of chiropractic care compared to medical care, and the authors concluded that their *review was unable to clarify whether chiropractic or medical care is more cost-effective.*

Essentially, this means that neither for chiropractic nor for homeopathy is there convincing evidence to show that the often-voiced 'value for money' claim is correct. As far as I know, there is no other form of SCAM where the situation has been shown to be different. In fact, in 2006, my team assessed the UK data for all SCAMs, and we concluded that *the limited data available indicate that the use of these therapies usually represents an additional cost to conventional treatment.*[16] I am not aware of any sound evidence that would require a revision of this verdict.

6.5. Alternative Cancer Cures

Imagine you consult your doctor and he says: 'I am so sorry, but I have bad news: the tests have shown that you have cancer.' You go home and feel as though someone has hit you with a sledge hammer. You cry a lot and your thoughts go round in circles. A complete nightmare unfolds; you sometimes

---

14   https://www.ncbi.nlm.nih.gov/pubmed/28915242.
15   https://www.ncbi.nlm.nih.gov/pubmed/27487116.
16   https://www.ncbi.nlm.nih.gov/pubmed/17173105.

think you are dreaming but the frightful reality soon catches up with you.

A few days later, you have an appointment with the oncologist who talks you through the treatment plan. You feel there is no choice and you agree to it—of course you do; you want to survive. After the first chemotherapy, you lose your hair, your well-being, your dignity, your control and your patience. You start wondering whether there is not an alternative to this misery and investigate what else there is on offer.

By then, several well-wishers have mentioned to you that the conventional route is but one of many: there are, in fact, alternatives! You go on the internet and find not just a few, you find millions of websites promoting hundreds of SCAMs for cancer—anything from diets to herbal remedies, from homeopathy to energy-healing. Many of them are being promoted as cures for your specific cancer, and all are advertised as free of those nasty side effects which currently make your life hell.

Who wouldn't be tempted by these options promoted in the most glorious terms? Who wouldn't begin to distrust the oncologist who kindly but firmly insists that 'alternative cancer cures' are bogus? Who wouldn't want to get rid of the cancer and the side effects in one genial master stroke?

Cancer patients yearn for hope and are thus extremely vulnerable to quackery. I do not know one who, faced with the diagnosis and all the misery it entails, has not given SCAM some serious consideration. Therefore, it would be extremely important that the information available to patients and their carers is accurate and responsible.

But sadly, it is not! In 2004, we assessed the quality of the websites advising patients on SCAM for cancer.[17] For this purpose, we evaluated those 32 sites that were used most frequently by cancer patients. Our results were shocking: many of these sites were of deplorable quality and most of them recommended a plethora of unproven treatments, most

---

[17]   https://www.ncbi.nlm.nih.gov/pubmed/15111340.

frequently herbal remedies, diets and mind–body therapies. Several were outright dangerous and had the potential to harm patients.

The consequences can be dire; you don't need to believe me but take it from someone who has the first-hand experience: *In 10 years of being an oncologist I have witnessed some devastating consequences when practitioners recommend 'alternative' therapies. The emaciated breast cancer patient who was told to present to emergency because there was nothing else her alternative provider could do to help her walk. Neither could we. She died of spinal cord compression after vigorous manipulation of her back. The man whose finances and prostate cancer had both spiraled out of control by the time he forked out $50,000 dollars on vitamin infusions. He regretted forgoing the proven benefit of chemotherapy. There was the man whose wife discovered the extent of his natural therapy debt only after he died and was forced to sell the house. There were the children who quit studying to help pay for their father's imported exotic herbs sourced from the wild. These stories are not unique – every oncologist tells a tale of financial and psychological ruin, experienced by the family long after the patient dies.*[18]

The level of misinformation in this area is sickening. Patients are being sold false hope by the truck-load. Yet they deserve better; they should have up-to-date, factual and impartial information on their illness and the best treatment for it. What they get in the realm of SCAM is a total disgrace: commercially driven lies about 'treatments' which are not just unproven but which would, if used as instructed, hasten their death. Some types of SCAM have potential for improving patients' quality of life, but no SCAM can cure cancer.

The problem is by no means confined to the UK. Members of several German Heilpraktiker (see section 5.6) associations were invited to complete an online questionnaire.[19]

---

[18]   https://www.theguardian.com/commentisfree/2015/mar/03/what-do-doctors-say-to-alternative-therapists-when-a-patient-dies-nothing-we-never-talk?CMP=soc_567.

[19]   https://www.ncbi.nlm.nih.gov/pubmed/24613909.

Homeopathy was used by 45% of them, and 10% believed it to be an effective cancer treatment. Herbal therapy, vitamins, orthomolecular medicine, ordinal therapy, mistletoe preparations, acupuncture and cancer diets were used by more than 10% of the respondents. The authors concluded that *risks may arise from these CAM methods as non-medically trained practitioners partly believe them to be useful anticancer treatments. This may lead to the delay or even omission of effective therapies.*

If ever a curative cancer treatment emerged from SCAM that showed any promise at all, it would be very quickly investigated by scientists. And, if the results turned out to be positive, it would instantly be absorbed into mainstream oncology. The notion of an alternative cancer cure is therefore a contradiction in terms. It implies that oncologists would, in the face of immense suffering, reject a promising cure simply because it did not originate from their own ranks.

But don't get me wrong: some SCAMs might nevertheless have a role in oncology—not as curative treatments but as supportive or palliative therapies. The aim of supportive or palliative cancer care is not to cure the disease but to ease the suffering of cancer patients. According to my own research, promising evidence exists in this context, for instance, for:

- massage,[20]
- guided imagery,[21]
- co-enzyme Q10,[22]
- acupuncture,[23]
- relaxation therapies.[24]

Unfortunately, the majority of 'integrative' cancer centres employing SCAM seem to bother very little about the evidence; they tend to use almost any exotic mix of treatments regardless of whether they are backed by evidence or not. In the interest of

---

[20]   https://www.ncbi.nlm.nih.gov/pubmed/19148685.
[21]   https://www.ncbi.nlm.nih.gov/pubmed/15651053.
[22]   https://www.ncbi.nlm.nih.gov/pubmed/15514384.
[23]   https://www.ncbi.nlm.nih.gov/pubmed/11391600.
[24]   https://www.ncbi.nlm.nih.gov/pubmed/11391600.

patients, we need to spend the available resources in the most effective ways. Those who argue that a bit of Reiki or reflexology, for example, is useful—if only via a non-specific (placebo) effect—seem to forget that we do not require disproven therapies for patients to benefit from a placebo response.[25]

But why are SCAMs like Reiki or reflexology nevertheless used for cancer palliation? I sometimes wonder whether some oncologists' tolerance of SCAM is not an attempt to compensate for the many inadequacies within the routine service they offer their patients. Substandard care, unappetising food, insufficient pain control, lack of time, empathy and compassion as well as other problems undoubtedly exist in some cancer units. It might be tempting to assume that such deficiencies can be glossed over with or compensated by a little pampering from a reflexologist or Reiki master. And it might be easier to hire a few SCAM therapists for treating patients with agreeable yet ineffective interventions than to remedy the deficits that may exist in conventional care. But this strategy would, of course, be wrong, unethical and counter-productive. Empathy, sympathy, compassion and good care are core features of conventional care and must not be delegated to quacks.

6.6. SCAM Advice for Patients

Many consumers using SCAM do so because they have read or heard something positive about this or that therapy. In other words, the encouragement to try SCAM comes usually not from healthcare professionals but from newspapers, the internet, books or SCAM practitioners. In this section, I will discuss these four sources of information in turn.

Newspapers

No doubt, some journalists have written excellent, informative articles on SCAM (let me use this opportunity to congratulate them for the achievement). At the same time, it is indisputable

---

[25]   https://www.ncbi.nlm.nih.gov/pubmed/15737827.

that misleading journalism on SCAM continues to cause harm on a daily basis. A plethora of promotional articles masquerading as journalism misleads vulnerable people into making wrong therapeutic decisions. In some cases, this will only cost money, in other instances, it may well cost lives.

In 2000, we published an investigation[26] determining the frequency and tone of reporting on medical topics in daily newspapers in the UK and Germany. Eight major daily broadsheets (four German and four British) were assessed for medical articles on eight randomly chosen working days. All articles relating to medical topics were categorised according to subject, length and tone (critical, positive or neutral). A total of 256 newspaper articles were thus evaluated. We identified 80 articles on medicine in the German papers and 176 in the British. There were 4 articles on SCAM in the German and 26 in the UK newspapers. The tone of the UK articles was unanimously positive (100%), whereas most (75%) of the German articles on SCAM were critical. We concluded that, compared with German newspapers, British newspapers report more frequently on conventional medicine and generally have a more critical attitude.

But that was years ago and things may well have changed since then. In 2006, we therefore conducted another investigation[27] aimed at assessing UK newspapers' coverage of SCAM, this time specifically for cancer. We covered three-month periods in 2002, 2003 and 2004, and a total of 310 articles were included. The results showed that interest towards SCAM for cancer had been increasing (81 articles in 2002; 147 articles in 2004). The most frequently mentioned SCAMs were diets and supplements. Articles mainly focused on SCAM as possible cancer treatments (45%), and 53% of all treatments mentioned were not backed up by evidence. The tone of the articles was generally positive towards SCAM. Promotional articles increased over the year. Our conclusion: *UK national newspapers*

---

26   https://www.ncbi.nlm.nih.gov/pubmed/11202946.
27   https://www.ncbi.nlm.nih.gov/pubmed/16703334.

frequently publish articles on alternative medicine for cancer. Much of this information seems to be uncritical with a potential for misleading patients.

The internet

Most people start seeking advice on the internet when they are ill, and in the realm of SCAM, they find plenty. Currently, more than 50 million websites offer advice on SCAM. This begs the question whether such advice is reliable.

My team has conducted several research projects to study this issue, and invariably the answer was concerning. For instance, we found that much of the advice for cancer patients provided over the internet would hasten their death, if followed.[28] Similarly, we demonstrated that adhering to the advice offered by chiropractors via the internet would seriously harm many patients.[29]

Perhaps this is best illustrated by providing a concrete example. According to their own description, the 'Alternative Medicine Society' is a *global network of medical practitioners and contributors who scour the best research and findings from around the world to provide the best advice on alternative, holistic, natural and integrative medicines and treatments for free.* This organisation provides explicit advice on '*7 common diseases you can treat through natural medicine*'.[30] Here are a few excerpts (the numbers in brackets refer to my comments below).

High blood pressure/hypertension

High blood pressure, or hypertension, is a condition most of us are really familiar with. Defined as the elevation of blood pressure in systemic arteries, hypertension left untreated could lead to serious, possibly fatal complications such as strokes and heart attacks. Conventional treatments for hypertension usually include a cocktail of several drugs

---

28   https://www.ncbi.nlm.nih.gov/pubmed/12189540.
29   https://www.ncbi.nlm.nih.gov/pubmed/20389316.
30   http://alternativemedicinesociety.com/7-common-diseases-can-treat-natural-medicine/.

[1] consisting of vasodilators, alpha/beta blockers, and enzyme inhibitors. However, hypertension can be managed, and altogether avoided with the use of natural medicine. Alternative treatments involve lifestyle changes (e.g. intentionally working out, alcohol intake moderation), dietary measures (e.g. lowering salt intake, choosing healthier food options) [2], and natural medicine (e.g. garlic) [3].

Bronchitis

Bronchitis may be defined as the irritation, or swelling of the bronchial tubes connecting our nasal cavity to our lungs commonly cause by infections or certain allergens [4]. Patients with bronchitis typically deal with breathing difficulties, coughing spells, nasal congestion, and fever. There are usual prescriptions for bronchitis, but there are also very effective natural medicines available. Natural medicines include garlic, ginger, turmeric, eucalyptus, Echinacea, and honey [5]. These herbs may be prepared at home as tonics, tea, or taken as is, acting as anti-microbial agents for fighting off the infections [6].

Eczema

Eczema is also a skin condition resulting from allergic reactions which are typically observed as persistent rashes. The rashes are usually incredibly itchy, showing up in the most awkward places such as the inside of the knees and thighs. Thankfully, eczema can be managed by lifestyle measures (such as avoiding certain foods which elicit allergies [7]) — and natural medicine. These include herbal components such as sunflower seed oil, coconut oil, evening primrose oil and chamomile [8]. These natural medicines contain different active ingredients which are not only able to moisturize the affected skin, but are also able to reduce inflammation and soothe itchiness [9].

1. Conventional doctors start with lifestyle advice, if that is not successful, they prescribe a diuretic, and only if that does not work do they add a further drug.

2. This describes the conventional approach. Unfortunately, it often does not work because it is either not sufficiently effective, or the patient is non-compliant, or both.
3. Garlic is not very effective for hypertension.[31]
4. This is not a description of bronchitis but of asthma; bronchitis is usually caused by a bacterial infection.
5. None of these SCAMs have been shown by good evidence to be sufficiently effective.
6. SCAMs play only a very minor role in the effective management of bronchitis.
7. Such measures are conventional and require conventional allergy testing to be effective.
8. There is no good evidence to show that these therapies are effective.
9. SCAMs play only a very minor role in the effective management of eczema.

Books

Other common sources of advice are books. Amazon currently lists around 50,000 books providing advice on SCAM. Surely, we can trust books, or can we?

In 1998, we assessed the quality of books on SCAM.[32] We chose a random sample of six bestsellers all published in 1997, and we assessed their contents according to predefined criteria. The findings were sobering: the advice given in these volumes was frequently misleading, not based on good evidence and often inaccurate. If followed, it would have caused significant harm to patients.

In 2006, we conducted a similar investigation which we then reported in the first and second editions of our book *The*

---

[31] https://www.ncbi.nlm.nih.gov/pubmed/22895963.
[32] Int J Risk Safety Med 1998, 11: 209–215. [This article is not Medline-listed.]

Desktop Guide to Complementary and Alternative Medicine.[33] This time, we selected seven best-selling SCAM books and scrutinised them in much the same way. The results showed that almost every SCAM was recommended for almost every condition imaginable. There was no agreement between the different books which SCAM might be effective for which condition. Some treatments were even named as indications for a certain condition, while, in other books, they were listed as contra-indications for the same problem. A bewildering plethora of treatments was recommended for most conditions, for instance:

- addictions: 120 different SCAMs,
- arthritis: 131 different SCAMs,
- asthma: 119 different SCAMs,
- cancer: 133 different SCAMs.

This experience confirmed our suspicion that SCAM books are a major contributor to the misinformation in this area.

SCAM providers

Even the advice provided directly by those who should be the experts, the SCAM practitioners, seems frequently to be of extremely doubtful value. A survey[34] of more than 9,000 patients of UK non-medically trained acupuncturists showed that a considerable number had received advice from their therapists about prescribed medicines. Since these acupuncturists are not medically trained, they are not qualified to issue such advice and the advice given is likely to be misleading. In 2000, we directly asked the UK acupuncturists' advice about electro-acupuncture treatment for smoking cessation, a treatment which we previously had identified to be ineffective for this indication. The advice we received was

---

[33]   https://www.amazon.co.uk/d/cka/Desktop-Guide-Complementary-Alternative-Medicine-Evidence-Based-Approach/0723432074/ref=sr_1_4 ?s=books&ie=UTF8&qid=1499771747&sr=1-4&keywords=ernst+edzard.

[34]   https://www.ncbi.nlm.nih.gov/pubmed/?term=MacPherson%2C+Scullio n%2C+Thomas%2C+%26+Walters%2C.

frequently not based on current best evidence and some of it also raised serious safety concerns.[35]

Many chiropractors from the UK[36] and other countries[37] make unsustainable therapeutic claims on their websites. In 2002, at the height of the 'MMR scare' in Britain, we conducted a study[38] revealing that a sizeable proportion of UK chiropractors advised mothers against having the measles-mumps-rubella (MMR) jab for their children. A survey[39] of UK chiropractors demonstrated that an alarming percentage of UK chiropractors fail to provide advice about the risks of spinal manipulation before commencing treatment. As these risks are, in fact, considerable, this behaviour amounts to misinformation and a serious violation of medical ethics.

Encouraging evidence exists for some specific herbs in the treatment of some specific conditions. Yet, virtually no good evidence exists to suggest that the prescriptions of individualised herbal mixtures by traditional herbalists generate more good than harm.[40] Despite this lack of evidence, herbalists do not offer this information voluntarily to their patients. When we directly asked UK herbalists for advice on a clinical case, we found that it was 'misleading at best and dangerous at worst'.[41] In other words, many herbalists misinform their patients and the public about the value of their treatments.

Many non-medically trained homeopaths advise their clients against the immunisation of children. Instead, these practitioners often recommend using 'homeopathic vaccinations' for which no good evidence exists. For instance, the vice-

---

[35] Schmidt, K. & Ernst, E. Internet advice by acupuncturists — a risk factor for cardiovascular patients? Perfusion, 2002, 15: 44–50. [Article not Medline-listed.]

[36] https://www.ncbi.nlm.nih.gov/pubmed/?term=Ernst%2C+E.+2008.+chiropractic+for+children.

[37] https://www.ncbi.nlm.nih.gov/pubmed/20389316.

[38] https://www.ncbi.nlm.nih.gov/pubmed/12228144.

[39] https://www.ncbi.nlm.nih.gov/pubmed/?term=Langworthy+%26+le+Fleming.

[40] https://www.ncbi.nlm.nih.gov/pubmed/17916871.

[41] https://www.ncbi.nlm.nih.gov/pubmed/12017746.

chair of the board of directors of The Society of Homeopaths had a website with the following statements: *Homeopathic alternatives to children's immunisation are now available... Our clinic offers alternative immunisation programmes for the whole family.* Such statements amount to misinformation which puts children's health at risk.

Finally, it is worth mentioning an investigation[42] we conducted in 2009 evaluating the ethical codes of the following bodies:

- Association of Naturopathic Practitioners,
- Association of Traditional Chinese Medicine (UK),
- Ayurvedic Practitioners Association,
- British Acupuncture Council,
- Complementary and Natural Healthcare Council,
- European Herbal Practitioners Association,
- General Chiropractic Council,
- General Osteopathic Council,
- General Regulatory Council for Complementary Therapies,
- National Institute of Medical Herbalists,
- Register of Chinese Herbal Medicine,
- Society of Homeopaths,
- UK Healers,
- Unified Register of Herbal Practitioners.

The results showed that only the General Chiropractic Council, the General Osteopathic Council and the General Regulatory Council for Complementary Therapies obliged their members to adopt the generally accepted standards of evidence-based practice.

Vis-à-vis such a high level of misinformation, we have to ask: how can consumers protect themselves from misinformation? Using the concrete example of a bogus cancer cure, I suggest that patients and consumers use the following checklist.

---

[42] https://www.ncbi.nlm.nih.gov/pubmed/19770119.

- **Is the claim plausible?** As a rule of thumb, it is fair to say that if it sounds too good to be true, it probably is too good to be true. In 2004, several UK newspapers reported that an herbal mixture called Carctol had been discovered to be an efficacious and safe cancer cure. As we have discussed in the previous section, it is not plausible that any SCAM will ever emerge as a miracle cure for any condition, particularly a serious disease like cancer.

- **What is the evidence for the claim?** In the example of Carctol, the claim was based purely on one doctor apparently observing positive effects. One newspaper headline read: *I've seen herbal remedy make tumours disappear, says respected cancer doctor.*[43] This, however, is not evidence but mere anecdote (see section 2.1).

- **Who is behind the claim?** Faced with an important new health claim, one should always check who is behind it. Check out whether this person is reputable and free of conflicts of interest. An affiliation to a reputable university is usually more convincing than being a director of your own private health centre.

- **Where was the claim published?** The Carctol story had been published only in newspapers. Even today, there is only one Medline-listed publication on the subject. It is my own review of the evidence which, in 2004, concluded that *the claim that Carctol is of any benefit to cancer patients is not supported by scientific evidence.*[44] If important new therapeutic claims like 'therapy xy cures cancer' are reported in the popular media, it is worth checking where they were first published. It is unthinkable that such a claim is not made first in a proper, peer-reviewed article in a medical journal. Go on Medline, conduct a quick search, and

---

[43] http://www.telegraph.co.uk/technology/3334063/Ive-seen-herbal-remedy-make-tumours-disappear-says-respected-cancer-doctor.html.

[44] https://www.ncbi.nlm.nih.gov/pubmed/?term=carctol.

find out whether the new findings have been published. If the claim does not originate from peer-reviewed journals, there is good reason to be sceptical. If it has been published in a SCAM journal (see section 4.10), my advice is to take it with a pinch of salt.

- **Is there money involved?** In the case of Carctol, the costs were high. Many new treatments are expensive. So, excessive costs are not necessarily suspicious. Still, I advise you to be extra cautious in situations where there is the potential for someone to make a fast buck. Financial exploitation seems sadly rife in the realm of SCAM.

For many vulnerable patients, SCAM turns out to be a minefield. Critical thinking, asking a few probing questions and doing a bit of research might protect them from getting ripped off, or — more importantly — from getting harmed.

6.7. Charities

Consumers and patients tend to trust charities, many of us donate money to them, we think highly of the work they do and the advice they issue. And, why shouldn't we? After all, a charity is an organisation set up to provide help for those in need. Charities offer a valuable service to society. Many charities are dedicated to assisting patients with specific diseases, and patients tend to trust their advice. In return, governments give these organisations a special status whereby they do not need to pay tax on their income.

Many charities are active in the realm of SCAM, and the obvious question is, of course, whether that activity generates more good than harm. Charities could, for instance, advise the public according to the best evidence about SCAM. In this case, they would undoubtedly provide a valuable service. If, however, charities publish advice that is not based on good evidence or even promotes bogus treatments, their work might achieve the opposite.

One does not have to look far to find charities exhibiting an odd attitude towards SCAM. Take, for instance, YES TO LIFE!

On their website, they state: *We provide support, information and financial assistance to those with cancer seeking to pursue approaches that are currently unavailable on the NHS. We also run a series of educational seminars and workshops which are aimed at the general public who want to know more and practitioners working with people who have cancer.*[45]

The website also informs us about many SCAMs and directly or indirectly promotes them for the curative or supportive treatment of cancer. Below, I have selected three examples and copied below the respective summaries as published by YES TO LIFE! (the quotes in brackets are the verbatim conclusions from my published research on the respective SCAMs).

Carctol

Carctol is a relatively inexpensive product, specifically formulated to assist cells with damaged respiration, it is also a powerful antioxidant that targets free radicals, the cause of much cellular damage. It also acts to detoxify the system.

(*The claim that Carctol is of any benefit to cancer patients is not supported by scientific evidence.*[46])

Laetrile

Often given intravenously as part of a programme of Metabolic Therapy, Laetrile is a non-toxic extract of apricot kernels. The claimed mechanism of action that is broken down by enzymes found in cancer cells. Hydrogen cyanide, one of the products of this reaction then has a local toxic effect on the cells.

(*The claims that laetrile or amygdalin have beneficial effects for cancer patients are not currently supported by sound clinical data. There is a*

---

[45]   http://yestolife.org.uk/.
[46]   https://www.ncbi.nlm.nih.gov/pubmed/?term=ernst+e+carctol.

considerable risk of serious adverse effects from cyanide poisoning after laetrile or amygdalin, especially after oral ingestion. The risk–benefit balance of laetrile or amygdalin as a treatment for cancer is therefore unambiguously negative.[47])

Mistletoe

> Mistletoe therapy was developed as an adjunct to cancer treatment in Switzerland in 1917–20, in the collaboration between Dr I Wegman MD and Dr Rudolf Steiner PhD (1861–1925). Mistletoe extracts are typically administered by subcutaneous injection, often over many years. Mistletoe treatment improves quality of life, supports patients during recommended conventional cancer treatments and some studies show survival benefit. It is safe and has no adverse interactions with conventional cancer treatments.

(None of the methodologically stronger trials exhibited efficacy in terms of quality of life, survival or other outcome measures. Rigorous trials of mistletoe extracts fail to demonstrate efficacy of this therapy.[48])

Another charity that might raise eyebrows is Homeopathy Without Borders (HWB).[49] To get an impression about their activities, here are the projects that HWB list for 2013:

- We plan to train as many as 40 additional Homeopath Communautaires in 2013.
- We'll support the Homeopath Communautaires as they grow with study groups and ongoing clinical support provided by our volunteer homeopaths.
- The 2012 graduates of the Fundamentals program will become teachers, moving HWB toward achieving our vision of Haitians teaching Haitians.

---

[47] https://www.ncbi.nlm.nih.gov/pubmed/22071824.
[48] https://www.ncbi.nlm.nih.gov/pubmed/12949804.
[49] https://www.hwbna.org/.

- We hope to bring continuing homeopathic medical care to the people of Haiti, reaching nearly three times as many people as we did in 2012.
- We plan to initiate a training program in 2013 for Haitian midwives and birth attendants for homeopathic therapeutics in pregnancy, delivery and postpartum care.

David Shaw, senior research fellow, Institute for Biomedical Ethics, University of Basel, Switzerland, has published a comment[50] on HWB in the respected British Medical Journal where he described the activities of HWB as deeply unethical and concluded:

Despite Homeopaths Without Borders' claims to the contrary, 'homeopathic humanitarian help' is a contradiction in terms. Although providing food, water, and solace to people in areas affected by wars and natural disasters certainly constitutes valuable humanitarian work, any homeopathic treatment deceives patients into thinking they are receiving real treatment when they are not. Furthermore, training local people as homeopaths in affected areas amounts to exploiting vulnerable people to increase the reach of homeopathy. Much as an opportunistic infection can take hold when a person's immune system is weakened, so Homeopaths Without Borders strikes when a country is weakened by a disaster. However, infections are expunged once the immune system recovers but Homeopaths Without Borders' methods ensure that homeopathy persists in these countries long after the initial catastrophe has passed. Homeopathy is neither helpful nor humanitarian, and to claim otherwise to the victims of disasters amounts to exploitation of those in need of genuine aid.

Yes, there are many responsible charities; but, undeniably, there are also many issuing misleading or irresponsible advice

---

[50]   http://www.bmj.com/content/347/bmj.f5448.

on SCAM. There is no doubt, in my view, that they can do much harm.

6.8. Great Expectations

Considering the many problems and serious concerns, such as the lack of efficacy and the risks of SCAM, it is most surprising to see that so many people use it. In this section, I will briefly discuss what patients hope for when they try SCAM.

Many surveys have addressed this question. In 2011, I therefore published a systematic review aimed at summarising the evidence from such investigations, entitled 'Great Expectations: What do patients using SCAM hope for?'[51] Seventy-three articles met our inclusion criteria. A wide range of expectations emerged from these studies [Box 14].

Box 15
The expectations of people using
SCAM in order of prevalence

- Hope to influence the natural history of the disease;
- disease prevention and health/general well-being promotion;
- fewer side effects;
- being in control over one's health;
- symptom relief; boosting the immune system;
- emotional support;
- holistic care;
- improving quality of life;
- relief of side effects of conventional medicine;
- good therapeutic relationship;
- obtaining information;
- coping better with illness;
- supporting the natural healing process;
- availability of treatment.

Despite the abundance of investigations included in our review, we concluded that *the expectations of SCAM users are currently not rigorously investigated.* The reason for this caution was firstly that most of the surveys were far from rigorous, and

---

[51]   https://www.ncbi.nlm.nih.gov/pubmed/21766898.

secondly that the research question seemed too broad to be answerable confidently.

The truth is that there cannot be one uniform set of expectations when using SCAM. The expectations will depend on a wide range of factors:

- The condition of the patient.
- The severity of the symptoms.
- The age of the patient.
- The gender of the patient.
- The patient's background, education, social status, etc.
- The patient's country of origin.
- The type of SCAM that is being used.

This means that patients' expectations are too diverse and personal to define in such general terms. It would be easier to name the reasons why patients and consumers are tempted or motivated to try a given SCAM in the first place. Many of them have been mentioned in previous sections:

- Patients might be dissatisfied with the many deficits of conventional medicine.
- People are bombarded with misinformation about SCAM.
- Many people have enough cash in their pockets to try just about anything.
- Some patients are desperate and would try any therapy that promises a cure.
- Many consumers are attracted by all things alternative.
- Some people are impressed by celebrities using SCAM.
- Many patients do not care about evidence but merely look for a compassionate therapeutic relationship.

Whatever the reasons may be, it can be helpful to understand what drives patients to try SCAM. If nothing else, this might help us to improve the offerings of conventional medicine and prevent people from getting harmed by charlatans.

Chapter 7

The Funny Side

I think the next best thing to solving a problem is finding some humor in it. – Frank A. Clark

7.1. How to Become a Charlatan

If you can't beat them, join them, they say. Quackery cannot be defeated; it will always survive. So, you might as well join them and become a charlatan yourself. At the very least, this might improve your financial situation considerably. To achieve this aim, I suggest a straightforward, step by step approach.

1. Invent an attractive SCAM

Did I just claim this would be 'straightforward'? Sorry, the first step isn't that simple after all. Most of the best ideas turn out to be already taken: ear candles, homeopathy, aura massage, energy healing, urine-therapy, chiropractic, etc. As a top charlatan, you would probably want your very own SCAM. So, you will have to think of a new concept.

Something truly 'far out' would be ideal, like claiming the ear is a map of the human body which allows you to treat all diseases by sticking something into specific areas of the ear — oops, this territory is already occupied by the ear acupuncturists. How about postulating that you have supernatural powers which enable you to send 'healing energy' into patients' bodies so that they can repair themselves? No good either, I'm afraid; Reiki-healers might accuse you of plagiarism.

But you get the gist, I hope. With a bit of dedication and some inspiration, you will be able to invent something brilliant, irresistible and highly profitable.

2. Find a good name

When you have identified your perfect SCAM, give it a memorable name. This is an important task: the name can make or break your new venture. Obviously, it ought to reflect the method you have developed. If it involves hitting your patient, 'slapping therapy' might go down well (sadly, it already exists). If you stick something in their ears and set fire to it, 'ear-candling' would be appropriate (also no longer available). If you put a garden hose up their unmentionable, 'colonic irrigation' seems fine (sorry, that one is not free either).

Do not despair; if all else fails, use your surname together with 'technique' — like Bowen Technique or Alexander Technique.

3. Invent a fascinating history

Having invented your treatment and thought of a sensational name, you now need a tantalising story to explain how it all came about. This task should be easy and might even turn out to be fun; you could think of something touching like

- you cured your moribund little sister at the age of 6 with your SCAM,
- or you received the inspiration in your dreams from an old aunt who had just died,
- or perhaps you want to create some religious connection — have you ever visited Lourdes?

There are no limits to your imagination; just make sure the story is gripping — one day, they might make a movie of it.

4. Add a hefty dose of pseudo-science

Like it or not, we live in an age where we cannot entirely exclude science from our considerations. At the very minimum, I recommend a little smattering of sciencey terminology. As you don't want to be found out, select something that only few experts understand; quantum physics, entanglement, chaos-theory and nanotechnology are all excellent options.

It might also look convincing to hint at the notion that:

- top scientists admire your concept,
- entire teams from universities in distant places are working on the mechanisms by which your SCAM works,
- the Nobel Prize committee has recently been alerted etc.

And do try to add a bit of high-tech to your SCAM; some shiny new apparatus with flashing lights and digital displays might be just the ticket. The apparatus can be otherwise empty — as long as it looks impressive, all is pukka.

5. Do not forget the ancient wisdom

With all this science — sorry, pseudo-science — you must at all times remain firmly grounded in tradition. Your treatment ought to be based on ancient wisdom which you have redis-covered, modified and perfected. I recommend mentioning that some of the oldest cultures on the planet have already been aware of the main pillars on which your SCAM today proudly stands. Anything that is ancient has stood the test of time — which is to say, your treatment has been proven to be both effective and safe.

6. Claim to have discovered a panacea

To maximise your income, you want to have as many custo-mers as possible. It would therefore be unwise to focus your endeavours on just one or two conditions. Commercially, it is much better to affirm in no uncertain terms that your SCAM is a cure for everything, a panacea. Your SCAM should be pro-moted as a cure for:

- acne,
- zooster,

- and everything in between the index of a major medical dictionary.

Do not worry about the implausibility of such claims. In the realm of SCAM, it is perfectly acceptable, even necessary, to be outlandish.

7. Deal with the sceptics

It is depressing, I know, but even the most exceptionally gifted charlatan is bound to attract these notorious doubters. They tend to be well-organised and frightfully switched on. Sceptics will sooner or later pester you for evidence; in fact, they are obsessed by it. But do not panic—this is by no means as threatening as it might seem. The obvious solution is to provide testimonial after testimonial.

You need a nifty website where satisfied customers report impressive stories about how your SCAM saved their lives, cured their children, improved their sex-lives, etc., etc. In case you do not know such customers, invent them—in SCAM, there is a time-honoured tradition of writing your own testimonials. Nobody will be able to tell!

8. Cheat with statistics

Some of the most hard-nosed sceptics might not be impressed with your effort of publishing testimonials. When they start criticising your 'evidence', you might need to go the extra mile. Providing statistics is an excellent way of keeping them at bay, at least for a while. The consensus amongst charlatans is that about 70% of their patients experience remarkable benefit from whatever SCAM they throw at them. So, my advice is to do a little better and cite a case series of at least 5,000 patients of whom 76.5% showed significant improvements.

What, you don't have such case series? Don't be daft, be inventive!

9. Play the conspiracy card

Focus on your ideal group of patients; they are affluent, had a decent education (evidently without much success), and are middle-aged and gullible, as well as alternative to the core. Think of Prince Charles! Once you have empathised with this mind-set, it is obvious that you can profitably plug into the persecution complex which haunts many of these people.

A straightforward way of achieving this is to rely on conspiracy theories. By far the best is to claim that Big Pharma has got wind of your SCAM, is positively petrified of losing millions in revenue, and is thus doing all they can to supress it. Not only will this give you street cred with the lunatic fringe of society, it also provides a perfect explanation as to why your ground-breaking discovery has not been published in the top journals of medicine: the editors are all in the pocket of Big Pharma, of course.

10. Ask for money, much money

I have left the most important bit for last: never forget for one moment that your aim is to get rich! So, charge high fees, even extravagantly high ones. If your SCAM is a product that you should sell (e.g. via the internet, to escape the regulators), price it dearly; if it is a more of a hands-on therapy, charge heavy consultation fees and claim exclusivity; if it is a teachable technique, start training other therapists at exorbitant fees and ask for a franchise-cut of their future earnings.

Over-charging outrageously is your best chance of getting well-known—have you ever heard of a charlatan famous for being reasonably priced? It will also get rid of the riff-raff you don't want to see in your surgery. Poor people might be even ill! No, you don't want them; you want the 'stupidly rich and worried well' who can afford to see a real doctor when things should go wrong.

Now you should be all set. However, just to be on the safe side and to prevent you from stumbling at the first hurdle, here are some handy answers to the questions you will inevitably receive from doubters. If voiced in public, these answers will ensure that the general opinion is on your side—and that is, of course, paramount in the SCAM business.

Q: **Your treatment can cause considerable harm; do you find that acceptable?**

A: Harm? Do you know what you are talking about? Obviously not! Every year, hundreds of thousands die because of the medicine they received from mainstream doctors. This is what I call harm!

Q: **Experts say that your treatment is scientifically implausible, what is your response?**

A: There are many things science cannot yet explain and many things that we will never understand on a scientific level. Numerous treatments used by conventional doctors are also not fully understood—or can you explain to me how paracetamol works? In any case, there are many ways of knowing, and science is but one of them.

Q: **Where are the controlled trials to back up your claims?**

A: The top methodologists now agree that clinical trials are of very limited value; they are far too small, frequently biased and never depict the real-life situation. Therefore, many experts now argue for better ways of showing the value of medical interventions. It is high time we finally abandon the obsolete paradigm of Newtonian science.

Q: **A highly-respected professor recently said that your therapy is unproven, is that true?**

A: This man cannot be trusted; he is known to be in the pocket of the pharmaceutical industry! He would say that, wouldn't he? Anyway, did you know that only 15% of conventional therapies are actually evidence-based?

Q: **Why is your treatment so expensive?**

A: Years of training, a full research programme, constant audits, compliance with regulations, and a large team of co-workers—do you think that all of this comes free? Personally, I would treat all my patients for free—and often do so, by the way—but I have responsibilities to others, you know.

7.2. Monty Python and the Homeopaths

Mercury is, as we all know, highly poisonous. It is therefore not normally allowed as an ingredient of medicines. Yet, many homeopathic preparations are based on mercury, as this text, for instance, explains: *The homeopathic remedy Mercurius corrosivus (merc. cor.) is prepared chemically using mercuric chloride and is used to cure various types of ulcers, especially ulcerative colitis (persistent ulceration in the large intestine). In effect, the common actions of the homeopathic remedy Mercurius corrosivus are basically similar to that of any other medicinal preparations with mercury, but it still presents its individual strangeness that cannot be found in any other mercurial preparation.*[1]

Regulators can't be pleased about homeopaths' frequent use of this poisonous heavy metal. The special plea of homeopathic manufacturers, therefore, is for an exemption from the law which would be required to allow the trade of homeopathic mercury remedies in future. In Germany, the homeopaths' lobby even had the support of some health politicians favouring a mercury exemption for homeopathic medicines. After some wrangling, a meeting of the EU committee on public health was scheduled to discuss the matter.

The following dialogue between the EU officials (EU) and the lobbyists of the homeopathic industry (LOHI) is, of course, entirely fictitious, but amusing and perhaps even reminiscent of scenes from Monty Python:

> EU: We are very sorry but, because of the undeniable toxicity of mercury, we will no longer be able to allow you to market preparations based on mercury.
>
> LOHI: But we have used it for 200 years, and nobody has ever come to harm.
>
> EU: We cannot know that for sure, and in the interest of patient safety we must be strict.

---

[1]   http://www.herbs2000.com/homeopathy/merc.htm.

LOHI: We appreciate your concern, but our remedies contain only very, very tiny amounts of mercury; they cannot possibly cause any harm.

EU: Sorry, but the law is the law! There cannot be any double standards in medicines regulation.

LOHI: To tell you the truth, our products are so dilute that they do not contain a single molecule of the ingredient printed on the bottle.

EU: That's interesting! Are you sure?

LOHI: Yes, absolutely!

EU: In that case, your remedies must be fraudulent, and we will have to ban them.

LOHI: No, no, no—you don't understand. We potentise our medicines; this means that the ingredient which they no longer contain gets more and more powerful.

EU: Are you sure?

LOHI: Absolutely!

EU: In that case, we will have to ban not just your mercury products but all your remedies.

LOHI: But why?

EU: Because either science is right, and your remedies are fraudulent, or you are correct, and they are powerful and thus dangerous.

7.3. The Scam Lecture

During my years as a SCAM researcher, I must have given about a thousand lectures. Essentially, this means that I have made every mistake possible. What's more, I had to sit through many more talks that were even worse than my own. Therefore, I consider myself to be a highly qualified expert on how to deliver a truly diabolical SCAM lecture. If you follow my straightforward step by step guide, you too might one day succeed in becoming a 'SCAM lecturer from hell'.

1. Ask for a hefty fee. This will impress the organisers and persuade them of your high calibre; more importantly, it will keep your bank balance looking healthy.

2. In preparing for your SCAM lecture, it is best to be cool and leave things to the last minute. Remember: you are so gifted and competent that a few scribbles made on the way to the venue will easily suffice.

3. Don't bother enquiring as to whom you will be lecturing to; what you have to say will capture the attention of a lay audience as much as that of a highly specialised one.

4. Arrive 15 minutes late! This little trick heightens the excitement of the organisers and the receptiveness of the audience.

5. The organisers might have suggested a topic. Don't get bogged down by such pettiness; you know best what you can lecture about. After all, it is always best to stick to what you know.

6. From the outset, you need to show the audience that you are better than they are. An effective way of achieving this aim is to display your knowledge of as many acronyms as possible. Making abundant use of abbreviations has the added advantage that it hides most of the glitches in your arguments.

7. Another golden rule is to never produce evidence for your statements. Some people use visual aids to display the evidence. This is both tiring and confusing, and it would, of course, require much more preparation than you allowed for. If you want to use visual aids, use photographs of your kids (pets, if you are childless) or your last holiday destination. This will add the type of personal touch that people adore. Surely, if they had wanted evidence they would have gone to a library and not to your lecture.

8. Spend as much time as possible with lengthy preliminaries, particularly if you are not really covering the subject printed in the programme. Mention, for instance, that you first met Cathy (the kind woman who just introduced you) when you were both in kindergarten and give a full and colourful account of your relationship since then. If you haven't actually been to kindergarten with Cathy, perhaps you

could talk about the car accident you witnessed yesterday and what it made you think of.

9. Alternatively, you could take the 'holistic approach', ask everyone to stand up, do a few relaxation exercises and feel the flow of energy in the body, room, or universe. The obvious aim is to leave as little time as possible for the lecture itself. Thus, you can pretend to know much more about your subject than you had time to disclose and you can end your unfinished lecture with the upbeat exclamation, 'Yeah! Perhaps another time'.

10. They will have given you a time limit for your lecture — ignore it! Only amateurs feel bound by such bourgeois constraints.

11. The discussion period after a lecture is the most challenging part of any presentation. But you're ready for this! You have wisely ensured that there is no time left for embarrassment. Thus, the discussion slot will either be completely cancelled, or it will be refreshingly brief.

12. Nevertheless, should a difficult question come your way, remember the important principle: you are so much cleverer than anyone else. And you must show it! Arrogance has always been a perfect shield for hiding incompetence.

13. A very good strategy is to ridicule anyone who dares ask awkward questions. Thus, they end up with egg on their faces instead of you.

14. In case, you don't want to be that mean, you could use the method perfected by politicians: ignore the question and come out with a lengthy statement that has nothing whatsoever to do with it.

15. If all else fails and you really don't know how to answer, a time-tested approach is to say: 'this is a bit complex right now; perhaps I could explain it to you over coffee.'

16. Make sure that you collect your fee swiftly and are safely on the way home when the coffee break starts. You don't want to communicate too intimately with your audience, in case

they find out that you're not quite as clever as you pretended to be.

The overriding principles of a truly diabolical talk are quite simple. Lectures are neither the time nor place for transmitting information and knowledge to those who came to listen. Their primary purpose is to massage the lecturer's ego and their secondary aim is to increase his income. If you keep this in mind, you will stop worrying about things like evidence, structure and delivery and simply enjoy the outing.

7.4. How to Avoid Progress from Criticism

Nobody really likes criticism, I suppose. Yet most of us would probably agree that criticism often is a precondition for making progress. So, we tend to grind our teeth and listen to it, introspect and try to learn a lesson.

Not so in SCAM! It seems that apologists of SCAM have developed five distinct strategies to avoid progress that otherwise might come from criticism (of course, these strategies exist in other fields too but, in my experience, they are particularly well-implemented in SCAM).

Ignore

We could also call this method 'The Prince of Wales Technique of Avoiding Progress' because HRH is famous for making statements 'ex cathedra' without ever defending them, or facing his critics, or allowing others to directly challenge him. When one day, at a scientific meeting, he seemed to advocate the Gerson diet for cancer, for instance, Prof Baum challenged him in an open letter,[2] asking him to use his influence more wisely. Like with all other criticism directed at him, he decided to ignore it. This strategy is a safe bet for stalling progress, and it has the added advantage that it does not require you to do anything at all.

---

[2]   http://www.medicalnewstoday.com/releases/10532.php.

Bluff

This method needs a minimum of basic understanding of the issues at hand, and therefore it is a little more demanding. It consists of looking closely at the criticism and subsequently shooting holes in it. If you cannot find any, invent some. For instance, you might state that your critic misquoted the evidence. Very few people will bother to read up and understand the original data. You are therefore likely to get away even with obvious porkies. To beef up your response a bit, pretend that there is plenty of good evidence demonstrating exactly the opposite of what your critic has claimed. If asked to provide actual references or sources for your counter-claim, apply the previously-mentioned technique and ignore the comment.

Sue

This is an extreme variation of the bluff method. All you have to do is to find a good libel lawyer (try to find one of the 'no win, no fee' variety) and start proceedings against your critic. This method was used by the British Chiropractic Association when Simon Singh disclosed that they were 'happily promoting bogus treatments'.[3] But be careful! It has obvious risks, as the outcome of this particular libel action clearly demonstrates; the BCA lost the case, plenty of money and most of their reputation.[4]

Invalidate

A very popular method is to claim that the critic is not actually competent to criticise. An example might be the discussion following the publication of an excerpt from a book critical about chiropractic.[5] Some angry chiropractors argued that the

---

[3] https://www.theguardian.com/commentisfree/2008/apr/19/controversiesinscience-health.

[4] https://en.wikipedia.org/wiki/British_Chiropractic_Association_v_Singh.

[5] http://edzardernst.com/2013/10/twenty-things-most-chiropractors-wont-tell-you/.

author was a failed chiropractor who had an axe to grind and thus had no right to criticise chiropractic (*Preston H Long you are a disgrace to the chiropractic profession... take off your chiropractic hat, you don't deserve to wear it. YOU sir are a shame and a folly!!*). Of course, you need to be a bit simple to agree with this type of logic, but lots of people seem to be just that!

Blame

Even more popular is the blame-game. It involves arguing that 'yes, not all is rosy on your side of the fence, but things on the other side are much worse'. Before they dare to challenge you, they should sort out their own mess; and while it is not sorted, they must simply shut up. For instance, if the criticism is that chiropractors with their neck-manipulations have put hundreds of their patients into wheelchairs, you must point out that doctors with their nasty drugs are much worse (*Long discounts the multitudes that chiropractic has... saved from dangerous drugs and surgery. As far as risks of injury from seeing a chiropractor vs. medicine, all one needs to do is compare malpractice insurance rates to see that insurance carriers rate medicine as an exponentially more dangerous undertaking*).[6] Few lay people will realise that this is a fallacy and that the risks of any therapy must be seen in relation to its potential benefits.

Attack

When criticised, many people get annoyed; therefore one might forgive them calling their critic names which are not normally used in polite circles (*who is this idiot, who wouldn't know the first thing about chiropractic*[7]). *Ad hominem* attacks are often the last resort of apologists of SCAM. They therefore emerge with great regularity when they have run out of rational arguments. But one should always look on the bright side—even of personal

---

[6]   http://edzardernst.com/2013/10/twenty-things-most-chiropractors-wont-tell-you/.

[7]   http://edzardernst.com/2013/10/twenty-things-most-chiropractors-wont-tell-you/.

attacks: it is easy to see that they are mostly an admission of defeat.

7.5. Politicians on SCAM

Many experts have commented on the often-laughable naïvety of politicians when it comes to matters of science or medicine. Politicians tend to think in time intervals of one election to the next and are therefore concerned too much about getting re-elected and too little about long-term prospects. As SCAM is currently popular, this means that many politicians support SCAM in the hope of winning votes. Some have even become true believers in SCAM, a phenomenon that is by no means new, as this excerpt of a speech demonstrates:

> It is known that not just novel therapies but also traditional ones, such as homeopathy, suffer opposition and rejection by some doctors without having ever been subjected to serious tests. The doctor oversees medical treatment; he is thus responsible foremost for making sure all knowledge and all methods are employed for the benefit of public health... I ask the medical profession to consider even previously excluded therapies with an open mind. It is necessary that an unbiased evaluation takes place, not just of the theories but also of the clinical effectiveness of alternative medicine.
>
> More often than once has science, when it relied on theory alone, arrived at verdicts which later had to be over-turned — frequently this occurred only after extended periods of time, after progress had been hindered and most acclaimed pioneers had suffered serious injustice. I do not need to remind you of the doctor who, more than 100 years ago, in fighting puerperal fever, discovered sepsis and asepsis but was laughed at and ousted by his colleagues throughout his lifetime. Yet nobody would today deny that this knowledge is most relevant to medicine and that it belongs to the basis of medicine. Insightful doctors, some of whom famous, have, during the recent years, spoken openly about the crisis in medicine and the dead end that

health care has maneuvered itself into. It seems obvious that the solution is going in directions which embrace nature. Hardly any other form of science is so tightly bound to nature as is the science occupied with healing living creatures. The demand for holism is getting stronger and stronger, a general demand which has already been fruitful on the political level. For medicine, the challenge is to treat more than previously by influencing the whole organism when we aim to heal a diseased organ.

What arguably makes this speech (the translation is by me) curiously funny is its origin. It was given by Rudolf Hess on the occasion of the World Conference on Homeopathy 1937, in Berlin. Hess, at the time Hitler's deputy, was not the only Nazi leader to promote quackery; others like Heinrich Himmler were perhaps even worse (see section 4.6). They were besotted with integrative medicine, which the Nazis elected to call Neue Deutsche Heilkunde (see section 5.5).

Today, there is no shortage of similarly bizarre quotes from politicians. A recent article in the 'Navhind Times'[8] is an excellent reminder of this fact:

> ...Town and Country Planning Minister Vijai Sardesai, on Saturday, appealed to the homeopaths participating in the All-India Homoeopathic Scientific Seminar: 'If the historic seminar is able to find a conclusive solution to our most endemic issue (kidney disease), then we think it would do a big thing to the state government and the people of Goa as a whole. Given the failure of the conventional medicines, we now have the alternative homeopathic medicines... Sometimes conventional methods don't give you solutions. It requires alternative methods just like in politics. So in the medicine, when conventional methods fail and the clueless about issues affecting certain section of the population of the progressive state, homoeopathy is the answer,' he

---

8   http://www.navhindtimes.in/vijai-urges-homoeopaths-to-find-cure-for-canacona-kidney-disease/.

added. Sardesai further opined that homoeopathy 'understands the healing mechanism of the body and Goa has slowly accepted it. Today, Goa has AYUSH Minister in Sripad Naik. I am hopeful that the people of Goa will switch to homoeopathic from allopathic. We pledge fullest support to it,' he declared gaining applause from the doctors across the country.

In the UK, Peter Hain (Labour) is a campaigner for homeopathy and wants to see it widely used on the NHS. He was quoted as saying:

> I first came to know about homeopathy through my son who as a baby suffered from eczema. He had it a couple of years but with conventional treatment the eczema was getting progressively worse and at the age of four he also developed asthma. We turned to homeopathy out of desperation and were stunned with the positive results. Since then I have used homeopathy for a wide variety of illnesses, but I rely on arnica as it's excellent for treating the everyday bruises and shocks to the system we face. My view is that homeopathy and conventional medicines must remain side by side under the NHS to offer the best to patients.[9]

If you fail to find this amusing, you need remind yourself of the difference between evidence and experience (section 2.1) — or is it perhaps Perter Hain who needs such a reminder?

The UK politician with the longest track record of supporting SCAM is probably David Tredinnick (Conservative). In 2017, *The Hinkley Times* reported:[10]

> Alternative therapy advocate, David Tredinnick has called for greater self reliance as a way of reducing pressures on the NHS. Speaking on the BBC's regional Sunday Politics

---

9 http://www.walesonline.co.uk/news/health/peter-hain-im-backing-homeopathic-2053093.
10 http://www.hinckleytimes.net/news/local-news/bosworth-mp-suggests-homeopathy-cure-12741801.

Show he suggested people should take more responsibility for their own health, rather than relying on struggling services. He highlighted homeopathy as a way of treating ailments at home and said self-help could cut unnecessary trips to the GP. He also said people could avoid illness by not being overweight and taking exercise... During debate on the show about the current 'crisis' in health and social care he said: 'There are systems such as homeopathic remedies. Try it yourself before going to the doctor.'

Mr Tredinnick has always stood by his personal preferences for traditional therapies despite others disparaging his views. His recent remarks have sparked a response from Lib Dem Parliamentary spokesman Michael Mullaney. He said in the wake of the NHS facing cuts and closures, Mr Tredinnick was yet again showing he was out of touch. He added: 'It's dangerous for Mr Tredinnick, who is not properly medically trained, to use his platform as an MP to tell ill people to treat themselves with homeopathy, a treatment for which there is no medical proof that it works. He should stop talking about his quack theories and do his job representing the people of Hinckley and Bosworth, or otherwise he should resign as MP for he is totally failing to do his job of representing local people.'

Many people would be influenced in their therapeutic choices by politicians. And it is therefore not just odd and funny but also worrying that some politicians show themselves so overtly ignorant of the evidence on SCAM (and other health-related subjects). If they do not understand science and medicine, at least they could refrain from commenting on such subjects, one could argue.

7.6. Prince Charles on SCAM

No book on SCAM can be complete without honouring the work that The Prince of Wales has dedicated to this subject. As a youngster, Prince Charles went on a journey of 'spiritual discovery' which took him into the wilderness of northern

Kenya. His guru and guide was Laurens van der Post, who later was discovered to be a bit of a fantasist.[11]

In 1982, Charles was elected as President of the British Medical Association (BMA) and promptly challenged the medical orthodoxy by advocating SCAM. In a speech, the Prince lectured the medics: *Through the centuries healing has been practised by folk healers who are guided by traditional wisdom which sees illness as a disorder of the whole person, involving not only the patient's body, but his mind, his self-image, his dependence on the physical and social environment, as well as his relation to the cosmos.* The BMA officials were so impressed that they ordered a full report on SCAM. The fact that it turned out to be highly critical of SCAM might not have amused the Prince.

In 1993, Charles founded an institution which, after several name changes, ended up being called the 'Foundation for Integrated Health' (FIH).[12] It was closed in 2010 amidst allegations of money laundering and fraud.[13] Poor Charles was again not amused, I bet.

In 2000, Charles wrote an open letter to *The Times*[14] stating that:

> ...It makes good sense to evaluate complementary and alternative therapies. For one thing, since an estimated £1.6 billion is spent each year on them, then we want value for our money. The very popularity of the non-conventional approaches suggests that people are either dissatisfied with their orthodox treatment, or they find genuine relief in such therapies. Whatever the case, if they are proved to work, they should be made more widely available on the NHS... But there remains the cry from the medical establishment of

---

[11] https://www.theguardian.com/books/2001/sep/22/biography.artsandh
umanities.
[12] https://en.wikipedia.org/wiki/The_Prince%27s_Foundation_for_Integrate
d_Health.
[13] http://www.quackometer.net/blog/2010/04/police-investigate-the-
princes-foundation-for-integrated-health.html.
[14] http://www.chiro.org/alt_med_abstracts/FULL/Prince_Charles_Alternati
ve_Medicine.shtml.

'where's the proof?' — and clinical trials of the calibre that science demands cost money... The truth is that funding in the UK for research into complementary medicine is pitiful... So where can funding come from?... Figures from the department of complementary medicine at the University of Exeter show that less than 8p out of every £100 of NHS funds for medical research was spent on complementary medicine. In 1998–99 the Medical Research Council spent no money on it at all, and in 1999 only 0.05 per cent of the total research budget of UK medical charities went to this area...

This time, I was amused: Prince Charles citing my research — what an honour!

In 2004, Charles publicly supported the Gerson diet as a treatment for cancer, and, as mentioned previously, Prof Baum, one of the UK's most eminent oncologists, was invited to publish an open letter in the *British Medical Journal*: ...*Over the past 20 years I have treated thousands of patients with cancer and lost some dear friends and relatives to this dreaded disease... The power of my authority comes with knowledge built on 40 years of study and 25 years of active involvement in cancer research. Your power and authority rest on an accident of birth. I don't begrudge you that authority but I do beg you to exercise your power with extreme caution when advising patients with life-threatening diseases to embrace unproven therapies.*[15]

In 2005, the 'Smallwood Report',[16] which had been commissioned by Prince Charles and paid for by Dame Shirley Porter, stated that up to 480 million pounds could be saved, if one in ten family doctors offered homeopathy as an alternative to standard drugs for asthma. Savings of up to 3.5 billion pounds could be achieved by offering spinal manipulation rather than drugs to people with back pain. Because I had commented on this report, Prince Charles's first private

---

[15]   https://www.amazon.co.uk/Scientist-Wonderland-Searching-Finding-Trouble/dp/1845407776.
[16]   https://en.wikipedia.org/wiki/Smallwood_Report.

secretary asked my vice chancellor to investigate my activities. Even though I was found to be not guilty of any wrong-doing, all local support stopped, which eventually led to my early retirement. ITN later used this story in a film entitled 'The Meddling Prince'.[17]

In a 2006 speech,[18] Prince Charles told the World Health Organisation in Geneva that SCAM should have a more prominent place in healthcare and urged every country to come up with a plan to integrate conventional and alternative medicine into the mainstream.[19] *The Guardian* commented that *a rational society should resist populist calls for a retreat from science – even when they come from the heir to the throne,*[20] and British science struck back;[21] anticipating Prince Charles's sermon in Geneva, 13 of Britain's most eminent physicians and scientists (including the author of this book) wrote an open letter which expressed concern over the *ways in which unproven or disproved treatments are being encouraged for general use in Britain's National Health Service.* We also argued that *it would be highly irresponsible to embrace any medicine as though it were a matter of principle.*

In 2008, *The Times* published my letter suggesting the FIH withdraw two of their guides promoting SCAM. My argument was that *the majority of alternative therapies appear to be clinically ineffective, and many are downright dangerous.*[22]

In 2009, the Prince held talks with the Health Secretary to persuade him to introduce safeguards amid a crackdown by

---

17 http://www.channel4.com/news/articles/dispatches/charles+the+meddl ing+prince/282452.html.
18 http://the-health-gazette.com/536/uk-prince-charles-supports-alternative-medicine/.
19 http://the-health-gazette.com/536/uk-prince-charles-supports-alternative-medicine/.
20 https://www.theguardian.com/commentisfree/2006/may/24/monarchy. health.
21 http://www.fasebj.org/content/20/11/1755.full.
22 https://en.wikipedia.org/wiki/The_Prince%27s_Foundation_for_Integrate d_Health.

the EU that could prevent anyone who is not a registered
health practitioner from selling herbal remedies.[23]

Also in 2009, the Health Secretary wrote to the Prince
suggesting a meeting on the possibility of a study on integrating SCAM and conventional healthcare approaches in
England.[24] The Prince had written to Burnham's predecessor to
demand greater access to SCAM in the NHS and told him that
*despite waves of invective over the years from parts of the medical and
scientific establishment,* he continued to lobby *because I cannot bear
people suffering unnecessarily when a complementary approach could
make a real difference.* He opposed *large and threatened cuts* in the
funding of homeopathic hospitals and their possible closure
and complained of *what seems to amount to a recent 'anti-homeo-
pathic campaign'.*

In 2010, Charles publicly stated that he was proud to be
perceived as 'an enemy of the enlightenment'.[25] In the same
year, Charles published his book *Harmony,*[26] which is full of
praise for SCAM and even went as far as advocating
iridology.[27]

In 2013, Charles invited SCAM proponents from across the
world to India for a 'brain storm' and a subsequent conference.
The Prince wanted the experts *to collaborate and explore the
possibilities of integrating different systems of medicines and to better
the healthcare delivery globally,* one of the organisers stated.[28]

In 2014, BBC News told us that:

---

[23] http://www.telegraph.co.uk/news/health/news/6701717/Prince-
Charles-urges-government-to-protect-alternative-medicine.html.
[24] https://www.theguardian.com/uk-news/2015/jun/04/black-spider-
memos-prince-charles-lobbied-homeopathy-funding-nhs.
[25] http://www.telegraph.co.uk/news/uknews/theroyalfamily/7147870/Pri
nce-of-Wales-I-was-accused-of-being-enemy-of-the-Enlightenment.html.
[26] https://www.amazon.co.uk/Harmony-New-Way-Looking-World/dp/
0007348037/ref=sr_1_1?ie=UTF8&qid=1384092482&sr=8-1&keywords=
harmony+by+prince+Charles.
[27] http://edzardernst.com/2016/02/prince-charles-the-immense-value-of-
alternative-diagnostic-methods/.
[28] http://timesofindia.indiatimes.com/city/kochi/Prince-Charles-appeals-
for-medical-collaborations/articleshow/25607695.cms.

Prince Charles has been a well-known supporter of complementary medicine. According to a… former Labour cabinet
minister, Peter Hain, it was a topic they shared an interest
in. 'He had been constantly frustrated at his inability to
persuade any health ministers anywhere that that was a
good idea, and so he, as he once described it to me, found
me unique from this point of view, in being somebody that
actually agreed with him on this, and might want to deliver
it.' Mr Hain added: 'When I was Secretary of State for
Northern Ireland in 2005–7, he was delighted when I told
him that since I was running the place I could more or less
do what I wanted to do. I was able to introduce a trial for
complementary medicine on the NHS, and it had spectacu-
larly good results, that people's well-being and health was
vastly improved. And when he learnt about this he was
really enthusiastic and tried to persuade the Welsh government to do the same thing and the government in Whitehall
to do the same thing for England, but not successfully,'
added Mr Hain.[29]

In 2015, *The Guardian* obtained the infamous 'black spider
memos'[30] which revealed that Charles had repeatedly lobbied
politicians in favour of more SCAM, free for everyone on the
NHS.

In 2016, speaking at a global leaders' summit on anti-
microbial resistance, Prince Charles explained that he had
switched to organic farming on his estates because of the
growing threat from antibiotic resistance and that he now treats
his cattle with homeopathic remedies rather than conventional
medication.[31]

In 2017, Charles was reported to be creating a state-of-the-
art clinic to offer free 'holistic' care for patients referred by NHS

[29] http://www.bbc.co.uk/news/uk-politics-28066081.
[30] https://www.theguardian.com/uk-news/2015/jun/04/black-spider-
      memos-prince-charles-lobbied-homeopathy-funding-nhs.
[31] https://www.theguardian.com/lifeandstyle/2016/may/12/prince-
      charles-use-homeopathy-in-animals-to-cut-antibiotic-use.

doctors.[32] A conference on 'integrated' approaches to women's health at the mansion this autumn will explore homeopathy, reflexology and acupuncture.

The late Christopher Hitchens repeatedly commented on the Prince's passion for SCAM, and his words are, in my view, unsurpassable:

> We have known for a long time that Prince Charles' empty sails are so rigged as to be swelled by any passing waft or breeze of crankiness and cant. He fell for the fake anthropologist Laurens van der Post. He was bowled over by the charms of homeopathic medicine. He has been believably reported as saying that plants do better if you talk to them in a soothing and encouraging way... The heir to the throne seems to possess the ability to surround himself — perhaps by some mysterious ultramagnetic force? — with every moon-faced spoon-bender, shrub-flatterer, and water-diviner within range.[33]

7.7. The 'Knighthood Starvation Syndrome'

The Knighthood Starvation Syndrome (KSS) has been a medical enigma for decades. Sporadic cases have been noted as far back as the 1920s, but recent decades have seen an alarming proliferation of incidents; some UK experts even speak of an epidemic.

The epidemiology of the KSS is most peculiar: it is confined to the British Isles, particularly to large centres, and seems to affect almost exclusively alpha males who have climbed up to dizzy heights on the career ladder and who therefore think of themselves very highly. A risk factor seems to be attendance at public school, particularly Eton. For a while, this led experts to assume that the KSS was infectious by nature, but this turned out to be a red herring. Later, it was speculated that the KSS is a

---

[32]　http://www.dailymail.co.uk/news/article-4700224/Prince-Charles-opens-holistic-clinic-Dumfries-House.html.

[33]　http://www.goodreads.com/quotes/268075-so-this-is-where-all-the-vapid-talk-about-the.

genetic disorder because it seemed to run in families, but this hypothesis proved to be false as well.

In most cases, KSS seems to attack its victims in their prime. It usually remains unrecognised for many years; early signs of dormant KSS include name dropping, pomposity, and a general alignment with the views of the establishment, the ruling class or professional peers. Some experts claim that the dormant KSS is identical with the better-known 'Brown Nose Syndrome' or BNS.

Later stages of KSS are characterised by:

- a sudden and often surprising change of opinion on professional, ideological and other matters which re-align the diseased with the dominant view,
- an abnormal need for political correctness,
- an insatiable hunger for favourable mentions in the national press,
- a phobia related to rocking boats or blowing whistles,
- an urge to get involved in charitable work and/or high-profile committees of any type,
- and an increasing ruthlessness in pursuing one's personal goals under the guise of pursuing the 'common good'.

Experts who have studied KSS in much detail claim that some of the features of KSS are reminiscent of a classical degenerative disease of the central nervous system, where the patient is afflicted by a galloping loss of critical faculties and irresistible need to please those in high places.

Opinions are divided as to the root causes of KSS. Some psychiatrists claim it is due to early childhood maladaptation or bad potty-training, while most sexologists are convinced that it caused by a chronically unfulfilled sex life, and psychologists tend to believe it is a form of mid-life crisis that was not allowed to blossom in a timely fashion. Endocrinologists have identified various abnormalities regarding the levels of stress and sex hormones, nutritionists are discussing a lack of vitamin D in combination with an excess of red meat and fast food, and

ENT surgeons speculate that it is caused by the absence of tonsillectomy during adolescence.

Unsurprisingly, SCAM practitioners have developed their own theories, most of which are, however, frowned upon by the medical establishment.

- Chiropractors view KSS as the result of a subluxation at the atlas level and advocate spinal adjustments followed by life-long maintenance therapy.
- TCM-practitioners are suggesting that a blocked kidney-chi has led to a pathological dominance of yin-energy, a minor aberration which could easily be corrected by acupuncture along the appropriate meridian.
- Bach Flower enthusiasts speak of vibrations being out of tune and recommend an intensive cure with Rescue Remedy.
- Herbalists subscribe to the neurodegenerative nature of the syndrome and advocate high-dose Ginkgo biloba.
- Naturopaths are convinced that KSS is caused by toxins from the environment and suggest treating it with an intensive cure of detox in the form of colonic irrigation.
- And finally, homeopaths see KSS as the final poof of their miasma theory. The bad air of the executive floor has caused severe damage which can only be corrected by an in-depth homeopathic history and prolonged, individualized treatment with remedies of extremely high potency.

Despite these and other attempts of altering the natural history of KSS, it tends to progress gradually in predisposed individuals, and symptoms are likely to worsen significantly over time, often to the point that the poor victim becomes a public menace. So far, the only known, evidence-based cure is rather heroic and sadly not often available: the award of a knighthood.

Experts claim that the only effective preventive measure against KSS is a healthy dose of critical thinking, rationality and scepticism.

Postscript

Some people say that I am fighting a losing battle and insist that SCAM cannot be defeated. It will be around forever, they say.

I quite agree with the latter parts of this statement. Humans seem to need some degree of irrationality in their lives, and SCAM certainly offers plenty of that. Moreover, conventional medicine is never going be totally perfect. Therefore, disgruntled consumers will always search elsewhere, and many of them will then find SCAM.

However, I disagree with the first part of the above assumption: I did not write this book with the aim of fighting a battle against SCAM. I can even see several positive sides of SCAM. For instance, the current SCAM-boom might finally force conventional healthcare professionals to remember that time, compassion and empathy are some of their core values which cannot be delegated to others. Whatever the current popularity signifies, it is a poignant criticism of what is going on in conventional healthcare—and we would be ill-advised to ignore this criticism.

In the preface, I stated that my main aim in publishing this book was to stimulate my readers' ability to think critically about SCAM and healthcare generally. My book is therefore not a text against but as a plea for something. If reading it has, in fact, made some of my readers a little less gullible, it might not only prevent them from succumbing to the Knighthood Starvation Syndrome (see last chapter), more importantly, it could improve both their health and their bank balance.

Thank you for bearing with me.

Glossary

Abstract, as used in this book, means a summary of a scientific paper.

Acupuncture is a SCAM involving the insertion of needles into the skin and underlying tissues at specific points for therapeutic or preventative purposes. Traditional acupuncture is mainly based on Taoist philosophy. Western acupuncturists believe that acupuncture is based on neurophysiological concepts. The effectiveness of acupuncture is not proven.

Adjustment is the term chiropractors often use for spinal manipulations.

Adjuvant therapy is a treatment administered in addition to other interventions.

Adverse event is another word for side effect.

Alexander Technique is a SCAM that focuses on the patients' posture.

Anthroposophic medicine is a SCAM usually practised by doctors and based on the mystical concepts of Rudolf Steiner. Various treatments are employed by anthroposophic doctors, few of which are supported by sound evidence.

Aromatherapy is a SCAM that employs 'essential' oils, usually combined with gentle massage; less commonly the oils are applied via inhalation.

Bach Flower Remedies are based on his notion that all diseases are due to emotional imbalances which can be corrected with one of the 38 remedies. They are too highly diluted to contain sufficient amounts of active ingredients.

Bias is the term used to describe a systematic deviation from the truth. In research, bias can produce results that are wrong or misleading.

Blinding is a term used in controlled clinical trials to describe the fact that trial participants are masked as to the allocation of patients into experimental or control groups.

Bowen Technique is a SCAM that involves manual mobilisations by a therapist, called 'Bowen moves', over muscles, tendons, nerves and fascia.

Case-report is a publication that includes all the relevant details of one single and typically remarkable clinical case.

Carctol is a herbal mixture developed by an Indian SCAM practitioner who has been promoting his remedy as a treatment of a wide range of conditions, including cancer.

Cherry-picking describes the habit of choosing evidence according to one's preconceived beliefs.

Chi (or qi) is a nebulous term for the vital energy that is assumed by TCM proponents to animate the body internally.

Chiropractic is a SCAM that was developed about 120 years ago by D.D. Palmer. The hallmark therapy of chiropractors is spinal manipulation which, they believe, is necessary to adjust 'subluxations'.

Chronic condition is a disease or symptom that has lasted for several, usually three or more, months.

Clinician is a healthcare professional—conventional or alternative—who looks after patients.

Clinical outcome is the term used for quantifying the results of clinical trials or studies.

Cognitive-Behavioural Therapy (CBT) is a form of psychotherapy combining cognitive with behaviour therapy by identifying faulty patterns of thinking, emotional response or behaviour and substituting them with desirable patterns of thinking, emotional response or behaviour.

Cognitive dissonance describes the conflict resulting from incongruous beliefs and attitudes or facts.

Colonic irrigation is a SCAM where enemas are given to flush out the content of the larger intestines.

Conditioning (or 'classical' or Pavlovian' conditioning) is a subconscious learning process where a certain response to a potent stimulus comes to be elicited in response to a previously neutral stimulus. This is achieved by repeatedly pairing the neutral stimulus with the potent stimulus.

Contra-indication is a condition that prevents or limits the use of a therapy.

Control group is the name of the group of patients in a controlled clinical trial that receive a treatment, often a placebo, to which the experimental therapy is being compared.

Controlled clinical trial is a study where patients are divided into two or more groups receiving different interventions the effects of which are being compared.

Correlation is a relation between phenomena or variables which occur in a way not expected based on chance alone.

Critical thinking (assessment, evaluation) is the process of conceptualising, applying, analysing, synthesising and/or evaluating information gathered by observation, experience, reflection, reasoning and/or communication.

Crystal healing is a SCAM that uses the alleged power of crystals to stimulate the self-healing properties of the body.

Cupping is a SCAM that originates from several cultures. Dry cupping involves one or more vacuum cups being applied over the intact skin; the vacuum is usually strong enough to cause bruising. In wet cupping, the skin is scratched prior to applying the vacuum which allows blood to be sucked into the cup.

Curative treatment is a therapy that cures the disease, as opposed to one that merely alleviates the symptoms.

Detox is an umbrella term for numerous SCAMs that allegedly rid the body of toxins.

Dogma is a notion put forth as authoritative without adequate grounds.

Double-blind is the term used in clinical trials to indicate that both the patient as well as the investigators do not know whether the patient has been allocated to the control or the experimental group.

Dowsing is a method of problem-solving that uses a motor automatism, amplified through a pendulum, divining rod or similar device. The best-known form of dowsing is probably water-divining, e.g. finding water wells with the help of a dowsing rod. In SCAM, dowsing is sometimes used as a diagnostic technique.

Effectiveness of a treatment refers to the clinical effects caused by the therapy (rather than by other phenomena such as the placebo effect) as demonstrated under real-life conditions.

Efficacy of a treatment refers to its clinical effects caused by the therapy under strictly controlled conditions (some treatments are efficacious but not effective; for instance, they might have significant adverse effects which overshadow their clinical effects under real life conditions).

Emotional Freedom Technique is a SCAM that is alleged to work by releasing blockages within the energy system which are thought to be the source of emotional intensity and discomfort. The treatment is similar to acupuncture but involves the use of fingertips rather than needles.

Empathy is the awareness of the feelings and emotions of other people. It is a key element of 'emotional intelligence' which connects oneself with others, because it is how we as individuals understand what others are experiencing as if we were feeling it ourselves.

Energy is the capacity to perform work and is measured in units of Joules. Energy exists in several forms such as heat, kinetic or mechanical energy, light, potential energy, electrical energy. In SCAM, the term is often applied to a patient's vital force as postulated by proponents of the long obsolete philosophy of vitalism.

Energy healing is an umbrella term for several SCAMs that rely on the use of 'energy', i.e. vital force; examples are Reiki, Therapeutic Touch and Johrei healing.

Evidence is the body of facts that leads to a given conclusion.

Evidence-based medicine (or EBM) is the integration of best research evidence with clinical expertise and patient values. It thus rests on three pillars: external evidence, ideally from systematic reviews, the clinician's experience, and the patient's preferences.

Fallacy is a commonly used argument that appears to be logical but, in fact, is erroneous.

Gerson therapy is a SCAM that includes a starvation diet of raw foodstuff and coffee enemas and is used mostly, but not exclusively, to treat cancer.

Heilpraktiker is a German non-medically trained SCAM practitioner.

Herbal medicine (or phytotherapy) is the medicinal use of preparations that contain exclusively plant material.

Homeopathy is a therapeutic method using substances whose effects, when administered to healthy subjects, correspond to the manifestations of the disorder in the individual patient.

Hypothesis is a proposed explanation for a phenomenon. To be scientific, it ought to be testable. Hypotheses are usually based on observations that cannot be satisfactorily explained with the currently existing scientific theories.

Individualised treatment is a therapy that is tailored not primarily to the diagnostic category but to the personal characteristics of a patient. Homeopaths, traditional herbalists, TCM and other SCAM practitioners individualise their treatments.

Iridology is a diagnostic method based on the belief that discolorations on specific spots of the iris of a patient provide diagnostic clues as to the health of organs.

Johrei healing is a form of energy healing that originated from Japan.

Laetrile (often also called Vitamin B17, although it is not a vitamin), is a partly man-made form of the natural substance amygdalin, found in raw nuts and the pips of some fruits, particularly apricot, or kernels. It is converted to cyanide in the body and often claimed to be an effective cancer therapy.

Lay practitioner is a clinician who has not been to medical school.

Life-force; see vital energy.

Manual therapies are treatments performed by a therapist with her hands; examples are chiropractic, massage, osteopathy, shiatzu or Bowen Technique.

Medline is the world's largest electronic database of medical articles.

Meta-analysis is a systematic review where the results of the included studies have been mathematically pooled to generate a new overall result.

Mind–body therapies are SCAMs which are thought to influence bodily functions via the mind.

Mistletoe (*viscum album*) is a SCAM from anthroposophical medicine based on the belief that, because mistletoe is a parasitic plant that can kill its host, it will also kill a cancerous tumour of a patient.

Natural history of a disease describes the progress of a medical condition when left untreated.

Naturopathy is a type of healthcare which employs what nature provides (e.g. herbal extracts, manual therapies, heat and cold, water and electricity) for stimulating the body's ability to heal itself.

Non-specific effects describe all phenomena which can determine the clinical outcome but are not due to the treatment *per se*. The best-known non-specific effect is the placebo effect.

Observational study is a non-experimental investigation, usually without a control group. In a typical observational study, patients receiving routine care are monitored as to the treatments administered and the outcomes observed.

Oncologist is a medically trained clinician with further formal qualifications as a cancer specialist.

Osteopathy is a manual therapy involving manipulation of the spine and other joints as well as mobilisation of soft tissues.

Outcome measure is the term often used for the parameter or end point employed in clinical studies for quantifying their result or outcome.

Palliative care is the treatment of patients aimed not at curing the disease but at improving their quality of life.

Panacea is a therapy that is effective for every condition or disease; such a treatment does not exist.

Pilot study is an investigation that is preliminary and typically aimed at determining whether a given protocol is feasible for testing a hypothesis.

Placebo is an inert treatment that has no effects *per se* but that can appear to be effective through the placebo effect which essentially relies on conditioning and expectations.

Plausibility relates to the question whether there are logical explanations for an observed or postulated phenomenon. The plausibility of a therapy depends on whether its mechanism of action is understandable in the light of established facts and science.

Pneumothorax is an injury of the outer lining of a lung which causes air to escape from the lung and renders breathing difficult.

Post-marketing surveillance describes the monitoring of adverse effects of a therapy while it is used by millions of patients. In conventional medicine, it is usually achieved by a reporting scheme which notifies the regulator of all observed problems in clinical practice. In SCAM, no effective post-marketing surveillance systems are in place.

Primary outcome measure is the specific outcome measure for which a clinical study was designed. Secondary outcome measures are usually recorded in addition.

Pseudo-science is a fake that imitates real science without having all of its qualities.

Phytotherapy; see herbal medicine.

Quality of life describes the state of well-being of a person. It can be measured by various means (e.g. validated question-naires such as the 'SF36') and is often used to monitor the success of SCAMs. It is frequently employed as an outcome measure in clinical trials.

Randomisation is used in controlled clinical trials; it means dividing the total group of participants into typically two subgroups purely by chance, e.g. throwing dice. The effect is that the two subgroups are comparable in all known and even unknown characteristics.

Randomised clinical trial (RCT) is a controlled clinical trial where patients are allocated to experimental or control groups by randomisation.

Reflexology is a SCAM employing manual pressure to specific areas of the body, usually the feet, which are claimed to correspond to internal organs, with a view to generating positive health effects.

Regression towards the mean is the phenomenon that, over time, extreme values tend to move towards less extreme values. Patients normally consult clinicians when they are in extreme situations (e.g. when they have much pain). Because of the regression towards the mean, they are likely to feel better the next time they see them. This change is regardless of the effects of any treatment they may have had. Regression towards the mean is therefore one of several phenomena that can make an ineffective therapy appear to be effective.

Reiki is a Japanese SCAM where the therapist claims to channel life energy into the patient's body which allegedly stimulates his self-healing abilities.

Sample size is the term used to describe the size of the group of individuals entered into a research study.

Sceptic is a person who habitually doubts notions which most other people view as established.

Science can be defined as the identification, description, observation, experimental investigation and theoretical explanation of phenomena. See also pseudo-science.

Shiatsu is a Japanese SCAM where the therapist uses his fingers to apply pressure to certain points of the body.

Significance is a term used in research in two different contexts. Statistical significance describes the likelihood by which a given research result is due to chance. Often it is expressed by providing a 'p-value', i.e. a measure of probability. A p-value of 0.05 indicating statistical significance means that chances are 5 in 100 that the result in question is due to chance. Clinical significance describes the likelihood by which a clinical result is important in a clinical context. For instance, a study might show that a homeopathic treatment has lowered systolic blood pressure by 3 mmHg; this could well be statistically significant but few experts would call it clinically significant.

Social desirability is the phenomenon that we tend to respond in accordance to social norms and in a way that we believe is expected from us.

Specific effect is the effect caused by a therapy *per se*, rather than by placebo or other non-specific effects.

Spinal manipulation is the term used for the manual adjustments of subluxations of the vertebrae often employed by chiropractors and osteopaths.

Subluxation as used in SCAM is an abnormality in the relative position of vertebrae which chiropractors claim to be able to adjust.

Symptomatic treatment is a treatment that alleviates symptoms without treating the cause of a condition.

Symptom score is a tool used in clinical research where several symptoms are rated and subsequently an overall score is created.

Systematic review is a critical evaluation of the totality of the available evidence related to a specific research question. Systematic reviews minimise the bias inherent in each single study.

Theory is the result of abstract thinking about generalised explanations of how nature works. A theory provides an explanatory framework for a set of observations. From the assumptions of the explanation follow several possible hypotheses that can be tested in order to provide evidence for or against the theory.

Therapeutic Touch is a form of energy healing where the therapist claims to channel life energy into the patient's body which is said to stimulate his/her self-healing abilities.

Traditional Chinese Medicine is a diagnostic and therapeutic system based on the Taoist philosophy of yin and yang. It includes SCAMs that emerged from China, including acupuncture, herbal medicine, tui-na (Chinese massage), tai chi and diet.

Vital energy is a metaphysical concept of a power that allegedly animates all organisms.

Vitalism is the metaphysical concept that life depends on a vital energy or force distinct from chemical, physical or other principles. The concept is found in many forms of SCAM, e.g. chi in China, pneuma in ancient Greece, and prana in India. The common denominator is the assumption that a metaphysical energy animates all living systems.

Yin and yang are to two opposing vital energies as understood in Traditional Chinese Medicine.

Index

CPSIA information can be obtained
at www.ICGtesting.com
Printed in the USA
BVHW07s1415180618
519329BV00004B/249/P